DEATH BY CIVILIZATION

International edition

Dr Peter Baratosy MBBS, FACNEM

Dr Peter Baratosy is a registered Medical Doctor in Australia. He graduated from the University of Adelaide Medical School in 1978. He is a Fellow of the Australasian College of Nutritional and Environmental Medicine and is an accredited Medical Acupuncturist with the Medical Board of Australia.

Published by Dr Peter Baratosy 2024

Original Cover Design Karen English

Modified by Nikola Boskovski

Edited Karen Mace

Formatting Nikola Boskovski

ISBN - 978-0-6451053-7-7 (print version)

978-0-6451053-8-4 (eBook version)

Dedicated to Jenny. Thank you for your support and encouragement. I could not have achieved this without you.

Table of Contents

PREFACE

In 1969, the song *"In the Year 2525"* by Zager and Evans reached No. 1 on the charts all over the world. The song warned of the dangers of progress, suggesting a future where mankind could be destroyed by its over-reliance on technology. The dates in the song may be all out of order and some things may have already happened, but the underlying theme is the critical issue: by relying more and more on these innovations, the necessities of life are being neglected.

This book has a similar theme; although I will focus on the diet and lifestyle that we have abandoned, rather than the technology *per se*. We are killing ourselves by **diseases of civilization:** ailments brought on by our neglect of the basics. This, unfortunately, is achieved by our brilliance, but also paradoxically, by our foolishness.

Undoubtedly, many wonderful, useful advancements have been made that have been a great boon to the world. However, it is not the purpose of this book to discuss these, or whether the good outweighs the bad, or vice versa.

> *"In every seed of good there is always a piece of bad."*
> **Marian Wright Edelman (1939 -)**

The innovations we have developed for ourselves have come at a price; however, we focus so much on these advancements, that we are neglecting the fundamentals of diet, exercise, sleep, and environment. We eat poorly, do not exercise, do not sleep enough, stress out too much, and live in a badly polluted world, which is a far cry from our ancestral conditions.

We are smart enough to know what we should be eating, but paradoxically, we are foolish enough to consume less favourable foods; processed foods with added colourings, flavourings, preservatives, sugar, including high fructose corn syrup (HFCS), and other chemicals which are non-nutritious and can possibly cause even more diseases. From here on, whenever sugar is mentioned, this will also include HFCS. HFCS is largely an American issue; it is only rarely used in Australia.

People eat in this fashion because, unfortunately, they are swayed by the advertising and, due to the busy lifestyle, there is a lack of time for proper cooking. Despite the multitude of cooking shows on TV, many people do not seem to know how to cook proper meals. It is much easier to get take-away food. Cheap, easy, and convenient, though not as nutritious as proper home cooked meals.

Most people's knowledge about nutrition comes from advertisements, produced by the manufacturers, to sell a product, not necessarily to teach proper nutrition.

This is a highly biased source. There is conflict of interest.

The underlying motive is profit and greed, not necessarily science.

We are smart enough to invent machines to do all our work, yet foolish enough to neglect our physical body and allow it to degenerate.

Will our species mutate into some other species, perhaps like the Daleks, that can only survive in their mechanical shells?

Our intellect has produced thousands of new chemicals, in line with the concept of *"better life through chemistry"*. Some of these chemicals have been useful, such as medicines, antibiotics, etc. yet, through our foolishness, we have abused and overused them without considering the ramifications for future health and wellbeing. There are other chemicals; harsh, nondegradable ("forever"), poisonous chemicals that are now doing us harm.

Our environment is being degraded at a faster and faster rate, which is having a drastic effect on our health.

We are the custodians of this planet for our children and our children's children, yet what sort of world will we leave them?

That is if we do have grandchildren.

We could be extinct by then.

Our technological brilliance is blinding us to the fundamental needs of our bodies, such as optimal nutrition, exercise, sleep and, even something as basic as sunshine.

It is this neglect of the basic needs of the body that is driving our species to extinction.

The human brain has evolved faster than human physiology. We will probably outsmart ourselves to extinction: we focus too much on what our brains can do at the expense of our physical and mental health needs.

The song, "In the Year 2525", predicts declining human health, declining fertility, worsening mental health, leading to the demise of mankind with perhaps a rebirth, a new start, sometime in the future: the figure of 10,000 years is forecasted.

I think the songwriter is possibly being too optimistic: I sometimes doubt if we would even reach the year 2525!

INTRODUCTION

Death by Civilization is a dramatic name for a book, The cover is also very powerful; and I will not apologise for that. I did this on purpose, as I needed a title that makes people stand up and take notice, a title that really gets into your face, because the topic I will discuss is so significant to the survival of humanity.

I choose to be controversial, perhaps even to frighten you. I don't do this for the sake of scaring you, but because I hope it will motivate you to do something with the knowledge you gain from reading this book.

Unfortunately, fear, though a great motivator, will achieve nothing in the long term. Knowledge, on the other hand, will enable you, and motivate you to make much needed changes.

Together, they could work even better!

> *"There are two levers for moving men ...*
> *interest and fear."*
> **Napoleon Bonaparte (1769-1821)**

There are many things I repeat, and I do this on purpose. Repetition reinforces and I hope it will reinforce my message. So, if you get bored, or annoyed, at seeing, or reading the same thing, then sit up and take notice. Ask yourself why this fact is being repeated.

Hopefully, this is a book that will motivate you enough that you will choose to start to do something; to help yourself, your family, and the people you love.

What is this big issue? Dramatic as it may sound, we may be talking about the demise of mankind. A demise that will come not from some outside source, a rogue asteroid hitting the earth, or nuclear holocaust, or pollution and global warming, or even alien invasion (though who knows, any of these may occur) but from something as simple as the way our body has reacted abnormally to the "civilized" diet and lifestyle we have adopted.

A major key is the hormone insulin, which will be discussed more in a future chapter.

Insulin is a normal, natural hormone, essential for

our survival. The problem, however, is that the unnatural western diet and lifestyle cause our bodies to over-secrete insulin, which in the long run can cause an insulin resistance (IR) and subsequent disease: **diseases of civilization**.

To some extent, saving ourselves from global warming, or blowing up a rogue asteroid or preventing an alien invasion, may be totally useless, if we wipe ourselves out anyway because of our diet and lifestyle.

We are dealing with a very serious condition and if something is not done soon, we could all become extinct. The sooner we start to make changes, the sooner things will improve. It will not happen overnight. It won't even happen in a few years. As you will see, the time frame can be measured in *generations.*

> *"The journey of a thousand miles begins with one step."*
> **Lao Tzu (flourished 6th century BCE)**

We are killing ourselves by civilization. We are killing ourselves by what we eat, by our lifestyle, as well as by the extreme stress we are exposed to. We are poisoning ourselves by the release of copious pollutants and chemicals into our atmosphere. It is going to be a fine line. Will we evolve (or adapt) quickly enough to this "civilized" eating and living pattern before it wipes us out? Only time will tell. Unfortunately, if we do not evolve to a different species, or, as an alternative, drastically change our diet and lifestyle, we may become extinct. In the stage before extinction, we will be a grossly unhealthy population with excessive mental health issues, and rampant with diseases of civilization that result in poor fertility, which would eventually lead to extinction anyway.

I hope I will be proven wrong.

You do not have to look too hard to see that this is already happening. The changes in our diet and our lifestyle have evolved faster than our genes and physiology can tolerate. We are genetically still Palaeolithic people, but we certainly do not live or eat like our Palaeolithic ancestors. Where we live, how we live, what we eat, how much we sleep, our quantity of exercise, our level of stress, our exposure to pollutants, even our exposure to sunshine, have changed and this all has a negative bearing on our health.

These changes to our diet and lifestyle are destroying us.

DEATH BY CIVILIZATION

I do not have to tell you how much dis-ease there is in today's world; it is self-evident.

The big question is "Why?"

I have alluded to the answer already.

Of course, the next important question is *"What can we do about it?"*

Hopefully, one of the reasons why you are reading this book is to make yourself aware of the issue and learn how you and your family can survive the **diseases of civilization**.

We are all becoming increasingly unhealthier. The rate of diseases such as diabetes, heart disease, obesity, cancer is all rising to unprecedented proportions - and these are all **diseases of civilization.**

Species can change in two ways: evolution and mutation.

Evolution is the process where species change, usually for the better due to some environmental alteration.

Mutation is another process where a species may change.

So, which is it? Evolution or mutation?

I believe those who favour mutation are on the right track, mainly because evolution generally produces an improvement in the species. Mutation, however, usually produces a decline in the overall health of a species.

We have changed from *Homo sapiens* to a mutant form: *Homo obesissimus.* Others have referred to this new species as *Homo stupidissimus.* (Have you seen the film *Idiocracy*?)

This is a very unhealthy species.

We are becoming fatter, dis-eased, unhealthier, and infertile, largely due to what we eat. It is also related to our sedentary lifestyle, our stress levels, lack of sleep and pollution.

So, the question we must ask ourselves is *"Why is our diet and lifestyle killing us?"*

The western diet is not based on what is the correct diet for the human species. Rather it is based on politics, commerce, and greed. We eat what the advertisements tell us to eat. A large portion of what we believe to be true about nutrition started in the offices of some advertisement company, and not necessarily in a scientific laboratory.

Many believe what these advertisements tell us. What is promoted to us is what the big multi-national companies believe will induce us to buy what they want to sell. Their concern is not our health, but their own profit.

Multi-national companies know what humans like: sugar or should I say, sweetness. So, it is no surprise that a large percentage of manufactured food has added sugar. Yet sugar is not a healthy thing to eat. People love it. It takes little advertising to encourage people to buy it, especially if it is touted as "healthy" or "natural". Much of the "food" is over-processed, essential nutrients are removed and synthetic substitutes added. Processed foods also contain colours, flavours, preservatives, and other chemicals which can add to the development of diseases. The companies make their profit, and humanity becomes increasingly unhealthy.

Drug companies then get involved, making drugs to "treat" these diseases. They are not necessary in collusion with the multi-national food corporations; perhaps a better term would be mutual parasitism.

We must make big changes to what we eat, and this should be based on what is healthy for the human species. If we eat properly, then we will not need the products of the drug companies so much.

Unfortunately, this will not happen easily because it will interfere with the profits of these huge multi-national corporations.

The answer is easy, but it will be very difficult to implement because of vested interests.

After reading this book and reflecting on what I have said, you can do something: vote with your feet. Do not go to the shops and buy foods which you know are bad for you.

If people do not buy these foods, they will rot on the shelves and eventually the shop keepers will not order them. If the shopkeepers do not order the unwanted products, in the end the manufacturers will stop making them. There is no profit in making something you cannot sell.

Of course, there are many "ifs" there, but one person, you, can make a difference.

Vote with your feet.

Another option is to ban unhealthy foods. In what are called 'the Prohibition years' (1920-1933) the USA tried to ban alcohol.

Were they successful?

No.

Alcohol went underground and there was criminal involvement. Banning or prohibiting something will not work.

Education will work.

The three worst foods in the present human diet are (not necessarily in any particular order) sugar, dairy and grains. I can now hear the howls of protest from the sugar farmers, the sugar refiners, the confectioners, the dairy farmers, the grain farmers, the grain mill owners, the bakers, the pastry cooks; yet all these foods are unhealthy. To ban these foods would bankrupt a large proportion of the country. This is where economics and politics come in. To do anything healthy would go against these big powerful rich industries. It will not happen for that reason.

Perhaps I am being too harsh; some of these foods I have mentioned may be taken in small amounts, on an occasional basis. And, yes, there are people who can eat these foods and not seem to be affected.

However, there are people who eat these foods and are not well. Rarely do they or their doctor connect their health issues with their diet, and particularly with the dairy, gluten, and sugar they consume.

The quantity of food consumed may also possibly be part of the problem.

So, if banning foods won't work, what will?

Only education and people voting with their feet will work; but it will take time and it will need mass action.

The human species evolved as a hunter-gatherer.

In the 21st century, we are still hunter-gatherers, at least from a genetic and physiological point of view, yet our "official sanctioned diet" does not reflect that. In fact, the sanctioned "politically correct" diet is probably killing us.

I want you to see why there is so much dis-ease in the community. If we have a close look, most chronic health problems occur in the developed world and in developing countries that adopt the western eating pattern. Yes, that is correct. I blame most, if not all our ill-health on high insulin levels caused by our diet and lifestyle. As you read further you will see why I am confident this is the case.

DISEASES OF CIVILIZATION

"If we could give every individual the right amount of nourishment and exercise, not too little and not too much, we would have found the safest way to health."
Hippocrates (c460 – c370 BCE)

Our modern civilization is killing us. This is largely because of our diet, lifestyle, and the stresses we are subject to, as well as the pollution that has been released onto our planet. Although we can only minimise the effects of pollution, we *can* do something about our diet and lifestyle.

Diseases, such as diabetes, obesity, heart disease and cancer, that in the past were rare or non-existent, are becoming rampant. These diseases, when they did develop, were seen predominantly in the elderly. Now we are seeing them in younger and younger age groups: and the frightening thing is that they are, to some extent, self-inflicted.

We are not living according to the genetic programme that is within us. We evolved, or perhaps I could say, we adapted to a certain diet and lifestyle over hundreds of thousands of years. This cannot be altered quickly. We are still genetically Palaeolithic people and therefore our diet and lifestyle must be in accordance with that.

But it is not.

Here lies the crux of the problem.

The western diet and lifestyle are virtually opposite to what our species had, in the past, adapted to.

Our paleolithic ancestors ate a diet higher in protein and fat and lower in carbohydrates and virtually no grains, refined processed foods, or sugar.

Today we eat excess sugars and refined carbohydrates: not to mention the added chemicals and preservatives.

Our ancestors led a very active life. Hunting and gathering is a very active existence.

Today we are mostly sedentary; we sit in our cars, behind a desk, in front of a computer and/or in front of the TV.

Our ancestors spent considerable time out in the sun. The sunlight on the skin produced vitamin D which is an extremely important substance. We evolved in the sun, not in a hole in the ground. Sunlight is a necessary part of our physiology and is essential for our wellbeing.

Today we spend most of our time indoors and when we do go out, we are sun paranoid. We cover up; wear hats and long sleeves and 30+ sunscreen. The "Slip, Slop, Slap" campaign is too efficient and has turned us into sun-paranoids.

For those overseas readers, the "Slip, Slop, Slap" campaign is an Australian Cancer Council Sun Smart programme designed to prevent skin cancer. Slip – slip on a t-shirt, Slop – slop on sunscreen, Slap – slap on a hat. This has been expanded – Seek - seek shade, Slide – slide on a pair of sunglasses.

Burstin and Allison, writing in the Adelaide *Advertiser* in 2006 describe vitamin D deficiency in children due to over-zealous sun protection. Of course, avoiding excess sunburn can protect our skin from developing skin cancer but the lack of vitamin D possibly can cause more bone disease, as well as breast, colon, and prostate cancers. The pendulum has swung too far the other way.

We woke up with the sun and went to sleep when the sun went down. This circadian rhythm and our health and physiology are all connected. Our health and physiology are connected to this circadian rhythm.

Now we are up till late at night, using artificial lighting to extend the hours we are awake. We do shift work which completely dysregulates our circadian rhythm. This extension of the light/dark cycle and the overall reduction in sleep is having drastic effects on our health.

Our ancestors lived in a relatively clean environment.

Today we live on an extremely polluted planet. Not only do we eat, drink, and breathe in chemicals that nature had never contemplated, we go even further by deliberately self-polluting our bodies by smoking and taking drugs, both legal and illegal, as well as applying all sorts of chemicals onto our skins. These chemicals and pollutants are influencing our health by producing disease, cancer and even affecting our fertility.

Of course, our ancestors were subject to stress. Daily living and finding food were stressful. However, the environment we now live in is one of continuous, and even extreme stress. We humans are also very good about worrying, stressing out over things that may never happen.

So, you can see that the diet, lifestyle, and environment our ancestors evolved with is totally different to the conditions we live under today. Of course, the environment our ancestors lived in was not all 'beer and skittles', it was hard and dangerous, but that is not the topic of this book.

Given the toxic environment of our world today, is it any wonder that we are developing unprecedented amounts of ill health that could lead to the demise of the human race?

Causes of death

People die. It goes without saying that we cannot live forever. We must die of something; however, the causes of death have been changing over the centuries.

Top causes of death in the Middle Ages.

1. Infant and child death (varied causes)
2. Tuberculosis
3. Fevers
4. Viral pulmonary infections
5. Diarrheal and GI infections
6. Malaria

7. Yersinia pestis (plague)
8. Childbirth
9. Strokes
10. Cancers
11. Rickets
12. Fractures
13. Mental illness
14. Scurvy
15. Famine
16. Dental disease
17. Leprosy
18. War
19. Gout
20. Social inequality

(https://www.researchgate.net/figure/Causes-of-mortality-in-England-top-20-causes-of-Years-of-Life-Lost-to-disease-1200-1500_tbl6_353013721 - Accessed 22 Jan 2024)

Top causes of death in 1850:

1. Tuberculosis
2. Dysentery/diarrhea
3. Cholera
4. Malaria
5. Typhoid Fever
6. Pneumonia
7. Diphtheria

8. Scarlet Fever
9. Meningitis

Top causes of death in 1900:

1. Pneumonia
2. Tuberculosis
3. Diarrhea
4. Heart disease
5. Stroke
6. Liver disease
7. Accidents
8. Cancer
9. Normal aging
10. Diphtheria

Top causes of death in 2000:

1. Heart disease
2. Cancer
3. Stroke
4. Lung disease
5. Accidents
6. Diabetes
7. Pneumonia/Influenza
8. Alzheimer's disease
9. Kidney disease

10. Blood poisoning

(https://www.attestationupdate.com/2010/10/21/10-leading-causes-of-death-in-1850-and-2000-2/ - Accessed 18 October 2023)

Top causes of death in 2020

1. Heart Disease
2. Cancer
3. Covid 19
4. Accidents
5. Stroke
6. Chronic lower respiratory disease
7. Alzheimer's disease
8. Diabetes
9. Influenza and pneumonia
10. Kidney disease

(https://www.medicalnewstoday.com › articles › death-statistics-by-cause-2020 – Accessed 19 October 2023)

Popular opinion is that cancer is now so rife because we live to a much older age. The presumption is that in the past, these people would have died at a younger age, of other causes, before developing cancer. This is not strictly true.

Many did die young. There was high infant mortality, many women died during childbirth and young children and men died of accidents or wars. There were famines and plagues that killed millions. However, those that survived to the age of 30 years had a life expectancy of another 30-32 years. This meant that those who survived to the age of 30 were likely to live into their 60s and above. Of course, longevity also depended on social class and region.

In the late 17th and early 18th centuries, approximately 10% of the population was over 60 years of age. So, we can say that there were plenty of elderly people living and not developing cancer but dying mainly of other causes.

Things have changed. No longer are we dying of mainly infectious diseases. However, infectious diseases are returning again, possibly due to the degradation of the immune system, which is caused by poor diet, poor lifestyle, and pollution. Also, people are now beginning to die from infections caused by antibiotic resistant "superbugs".

Overall, we are now dying more with diseases caused by civilization: chronic diseases which are largely caused by diet and lifestyle issues.

One cause of death not included in the above statistics is iatrogenic disease; disease caused by doctor's treatments and/or mistakes. Modern medicine has saved many lives but on the other side of the coin, has harmed many as well.

"Experts estimate that as many as 98,000 people die in any given year from medical errors that occur in hospitals. That's more than die from motor vehicle accidents, breast cancer, or AIDS ..."
(Kohn, Corrigan, & Donaldson (editors), 2000).

This is confirmed by Gøtzsche (2014) who noted that *"... prescription drugs are the third leading cause of death after heart disease and cancer ..."*

A more recent study by Makary and Daniel (2016) confirmed this.

Now that is a frightening statistic.

> *"The medical establishment has become a major threat to health."*
> **Ivan Illich (1926 – 2002)**

Other than the unusual situation with Covid, the top causes of death today are what we can call **diseases of civilization**, which as mentioned, are largely caused by faulty diet and lifestyle.

There is evidence that even Covid morbidity/mortality in many cases is related to lifestyle factors, such as obesity and vitamin D deficiency. Covid, then, can be included in **diseases of civilisation** (Gonçalves et al., 2020) since evidence demonstrates that morbidity/mortality can be minimised if not prevented.

People living in our modern western culture eat many foods that did not exist in the past. Notably, these are refined, "white" bread, sugars, pasta, and other refined carbohydrates, polyunsaturated oils, trans fatty acids, and other manufactured "foods" (I use inverted commas on purpose).

> *"Don't eat anything you great-great-great grandmother wouldn't recognise as food."*
> **Michael Pollan (1955 -)**

These so-called "foods" are what we now call "junk food". (Not real food!) A poor diet causes the increase in chronic diseases, which cause many deaths. What is even more frightening is that this high carbohydrate, low fat diet, is the officially sanctioned diet, a diet completely opposite to our ancestral diet.

This officially sanctioned diet is not based on science but on politics.

Many of the top causes of death, the **disease of civilization**, are related to metabolic syndrome and I will discuss and explore this as we proceed.

METABOLIC SYNDROME

"Before you heal someone, ask him if he's willing to give up the things that make him sick."
Hippocrates (c460 – c370 BCE)

This book is largely about metabolic syndrome (MetS), which in the past was known as "syndrome X". Syndrome X was first described by Gerald Reaven (1928 – 2018) in 1988. One of the underlying issues is the development of elevated levels of insulin in the blood (hyperinsulinaemia) with subsequent development of insulin resistance (IR). The excess insulin levels and the subsequent IR - cause a large proportion of the diseases in the western world; and I say the western world because, primitive, and/or less developed nations, eating their traditional diets and following their traditional lifestyle patterns, have virtually none of these health concerns. They may have other health problems but that is another issue.

According to Saklayen (2018) the incidence of MetS is about 25% of the world population, and this incidence will rise as the less developed nations adapt to a western style diet and lifestyle.

Noubiap et al. (2022) state that the incidence is between 12.5% to 31.4% of the world's population, depending on the definition used.

That is a lot of people.

The causes of most **diseases of civilization** are the modern western diet, and lifestyle. These encourage excess serum insulin levels, which leads to IR.

So, what is MetS?

Most have not heard about it, not even doctors, yet it is all around us. Some doctors have heard about it, but unfortunately believe it is a relatively rare and un-important condition. As we have seen, however, it is perhaps the most common condition in western society.

A syndrome is a condition defined by a cluster of related symptoms or disorders: in the case of MetS, the cluster of symptoms includes elevated blood sugar levels (diabetes), elevated weight (obesity), elevated blood pressure (hypertension) and elevated cholesterol levels (hypercholesterolaemia). Cancer can also be added to this list.

DEATH BY CIVILIZATION

Review the list of causes of death in 2020 in the previous chapter. Note that these conditions are near the top of the list, yet they are absent from the medieval and the 1850 lists. They are becoming more evident on the 1900 list.

Reflect on these conditions for a while: diabetes, obesity, hypertension, hypercholesterolaemia, cancer: these are all increasingly common problems found in modern western society.

Billions of dollars are spent on medical expenses to deal with these health problems. To some extent it could be said that this money is wasted because the money is being spent on looking only at the symptoms, the superficial manifestations. Dealing only with the superficial manifestations will not totally resolve the problem.

One of the fundamental principles in treatment of any illness or disease is to deal with the underlying condition. Correct the underlying problem and many of the symptoms may be resolved, and if treatment is started early enough, may be prevented.

While treating the underlying metabolism is essential, it is also absolutely necessary to deal with the superficial manifestations.

Many of these problems can be prevented by some very simple changes; the earlier the better.

These individual disorders have been known for a long time and have been treated as individual diseases or conditions, with varying degrees of success. Many are known to co-exist and only recently was the connection made that these conditions have a common underlying cause.

The underlying cause is a metabolic problem: a problem caused by something as essential as what we eat and how we live our lives. This underlying condition is known as hyperinsulinaemia, that is, excess insulin in the blood. This eventually results in IR, which means that the body becomes resistant or insensitive to the action of insulin. To understand the condition, we must understand the function of insulin, which is a very fundamental hormone. This will be explored later.

Many of these individual conditions were treated symptomatically only, and that is why the treatment was not optimal.

The underlying metabolic abnormality is hyperinsulinaemia (excess insulin) which leads to insulin resistance (IR).

Contrary to orthodox medical thinking, I purport that diabetes is not really a disease, but a symptom.

This can be said also for hypertension and for high cholesterol. These are not diseases: they are symptoms. A symptom of an underlying metabolic condition.

In diabetes, the aim of treatment is to lower the blood sugar level (BSL), in hypertension the treatment involves reducing the blood pressure (BP), in obesity and high cholesterol, treatment also involves "reducing the numbers", the weight or the cholesterol level. This is all just superficial symptomatic treatment. Symptomatic treatment, i.e. "reducing the numbers" can decrease morbidity and mortality to a certain extent but it is not the full answer.

This is possibly why treatment of the individual conditions has not been as effective as it should be, because only the symptoms were treated and not the underlying cause.

Treat the underlying metabolism but also treat the superficial manifestations.

Let us use the analogy of a car. Imagine we are

driving down the road and we see that the temperature gauge on the dashboard is showing hot. What do we do? Do we fiddle about with the gauge and make it show a lower temperature, or do we have a look under the bonnet and determine why the engine was overheating and repair the engine. Fiddling about with the temperature gauge will not make the engine run any cooler.

Just like the car, lowering the BSL, or BP will not necessarily improve health. We must treat the underlying problem. We must treat the underlying metabolism and not just "reduce the numbers", even though "lowering the numbers" does produce some benefit.

Diabetes is not a disease of blood sugar level. Therefore, just lowering the BSL does not necessarily give better health.

Does just lowering the BP reduce heart disease? As we shall see, no, just lowering BP does not necessarily improve health. Lowering of BP, however, can help prevent heart attacks or strokes, but there is more to it than that.

What about cholesterol? There is a great hype about cholesterol. Lower it or you will die, seems to be the current thinking. But is this correct?

Lowering cholesterol does not necessarily give better health or longer healthier lives. Like the temperature gauge, cholesterol is a marker and/or a risk factor.

Do we have to lower cholesterol *per se?* Or do we deal with what causes the cholesterol level to go up?

Yes, there are studies which show that lowering cholesterol with statin drugs does reduce heart disease. Though some of this is a clever trick, a statistical fiddle, expressing results as a relative outcome, rather than an absolute outcome.

To use an outrageous example, if, in a study, the placebo group had 2 episodes, while the drug group had 1 episode, in relative terms; there is a 50% reduction: and this is the figure that is advertised. In absolute terms, there is probably no statistical difference.

Don't forget that there is always a conflict of interest. Who did the study? Who paid for it? Was it done by a truly independent researcher?

Much of the research and many drug trials are paid for by the drug companies. Since they pay for it, they have a large say in what is published and what is not.

"He who pays the piper, calls the tune."

The drug companies design the study, sometimes even ghost-write the report which can have a profound effect on the results (Mlinarić, Horvat, & Šupak Smolčić, 2017).

The term "epistemic corruption" is used to describe the action of pharmaceutical companies on medical science. Sismondo (2021) wrote *"There is now abundant evidence that the involvement of pharmaceutical companies corrupts medical science."*

Drug trials financed by the drug companies show more positive results for their products than independent trials of the same product (Schott et al., 2010).

Some studies have shown that lowering cholesterol with statins can produce an improvement in heart disease, however, this is not necessarily caused by lowering the cholesterol *per se* but by some other action of these drugs. This will be discussed later.

In many cases, cholesterol levels do drop if the underlying metabolism is dealt with. It is important to note that cholesterol is a marker; it is not a disease *per se*. It is a marker of an underlying metabolic problem.

Risk factors are not diseases.

Obesity is a big problem (sorry about the pun). Losing weight will probably improve health. Gastric bypass surgery can cause weight loss but that will not necessarily change the underlying metabolism. It is important to understand that losing weight can only be achieved with a change in diet and lifestyle. By this, I mean a permanent change in diet and lifestyle: rather than a temporary change. Of course, anyone can lose weight with a strict, extreme diet but weight will return, with a vengeance, when you revert to old habits.

Drug companies release drugs that help a person to reduce weight. Although the person will lose weight, such drugs are expensive (good for profits) and probably unsafe. Generally, this is not a healthy way to lose weight and weight will return when the drugs are stopped. So, people will have to stay on these drugs. Yes, good for ongoing profit. Here again, we are just changing a number. The number on the scales. For healthy weight loss, we must change the underlying metabolism.

> Our metabolism is running in an abnormal fashion, in response to the abnormal conditions we are placing on our bodies.

The unfortunate thing is that this underlying metabolism that I have up until now mentioned many times is caused largely by our diet and lifestyle.

We don't have to be blind Freddy to see that the health of most people living in a western society is not good. In fact, it is terrible.

How common are these conditions?

Cordain, Eades, and Eades (2003) published the following figures, which are from the USA, and probably any western country will be similar. The figures are over 20 years old and are probably much worse now.

- 63% of men and 55% of women over age 25 are either overweight or obese.
- Estimated number of deaths ascribable to obesity is 280,184 per year.
- More than 60,000,000 Americans have one or more types of cardiovascular disease, which represents the leading cause of mortality (40.6% of all deaths).

- 50,000,000 Americans are hypertensive.
- 10,000,000 have type 2 diabetes (though I think the actual figure could be much higher).
- 72,000,000 have total cholesterol/HDL ratios of greater than 4.5.

The researchers concluded that *"Accordingly, diseases of insulin resistance represent far and away the major health problem, not just in the USA, but in virtually all of western civilization."*

What is the cause of all this disease? Could it be as simple as our diet and our unnatural lifestyle?

More than likely "yes".

We must go back to our distant past to see how this all develops. The human species had been hunter-gatherers for a very, very long time. A great deal of our species' evolution occurred during this time, and we can make a reasonable assumption that our physiology and digestion were adapted to this hunter-gatherer diet and lifestyle.

Approximately 10,000 years ago, things began to change. Agriculture and animal husbandry were introduced. This was probably a necessity as the population was growing and the number of wild animals for hunting had declined.

This change in diet had occurred too quickly for the human genome to adjust. (Cordain et al., 2005) (emphasis the author)

Evolution, or adaptation, occurs over generations: genetic and physiological changes mould to the environment and more importantly, to the diet. We cannot adapt to one diet over hundreds of thousands of years and then relatively suddenly change to a completely different diet.

This is, in fact, what has happened, and this is probably the cause of most of our problems.

Cordain et al. (2005) argue that during the neolithic and industrial periods, the human diet changed very radically in seven crucial aspects.

These seven differences are:

1. Glycaemic load
2. Fatty acid composition
3. Macronutrient composition
4. Micronutrient composition
5. Acid-base balance
6. Sodium-potassium ratio
7. Fibre content.

1. Glycaemic load

Over the centuries, human society moved from a hunter-gatherer existence to an agricultural diet and then, with the industrial revolution, even more changes were made to the food that we now eat.

The hunter-gatherers ate a diet of minimally processed animal foods and wild plants: estimated to be about 65% animal origin and 35% plant origin, although this varied from season to season and region to region. The coming of agriculture changed this diet to one which human physiology had not had experience with. Dairy and refined sugar were introduced, as was food such as grains which contain gluten. Initially, these were introduced slowly, but then with increasing rapidity. The per capita consumption of refined sucrose rose from 6.8 Kg in 1815 to 54.5 Kg in 1970.

We are now suffering from this diet. Our bodies have not adapted to this eating pattern.

"Although dairy products, cereals, refined sugars, refined vegetable oils and alcohol make up 72.1% of the total daily energy consumed by all people in the United States, these types of foods would have contributed little or none of the energy in the typical preagricultural hominin diet"
(Cordain et al., 2005).

2. Fatty acid composition

Our ancestors ate a fatty diet. They ate animal fats, though the content did vary between end of summer fat content and the beginning of spring content. Things changed when animal husbandry began. The aim was to keep higher fat contents in the animals for a longer, more consistent period, and this increased the overall fat intake.

Also, from the beginning of the 19th century, the use of vegetable oils greatly increased. Between 1909 and 1999, the per capita consumption of salad and cooking oils increased by 130%. This increase of refined vegetable oil altered the fat consumption of humans.

Another important change has been in the omega 3: omega 6 ratio. Our ancestral diet consisted of a higher omega 3 content, which produced an omega 3: omega 6 ratio of 1:1. The current western diet, with its reliance on plant oils and grains, produces an omega 3: omega 6 ratio of 1:40 or even higher.

Free-range, grass-fed animals and eggs from free-range chickens contain a more beneficial omega 3: omega 6 ratio.

Commercially farmed animals and chickens are fed a diet, usually based on grain, which is high in omega 6 and therefore the meat and the eggs have an altered omega 3: omega 6 ratio.

As we shall see, omega 3 fatty acids are integral in preventing the risk of chronic disease and promoting health, especially heart disease.

I should also mention *trans* fatty acids (TFAs) here. These are fatty acids that have been altered due to heating or due to processing. In humans, the fatty acids are in the *cis* isomer structure. A change to the *trans* structure has significant health issues. An oil, liquid at room temperature is hydrogenated to make it solid at room temperature, this product is margarine, a product that is high in TFAs.

3. Macronutrient composition

A macronutrient is defined as a nutrient required in large amounts for the normal growth of an organism and usually refers to: 1. proteins, 2. fats, and 3. carbohydrates.

The current USA diet, and there is no reason to believe that the current Australian diet is any different, consists of a mixture of these macronutrients: carbohydrates 51.8%, fat 32.8% and protein 15.4%. These proportions differ greatly from data gathered from hunter-gatherer societies, where the protein levels are much higher, and the carbohydrate levels are much lower. For obvious reasons, the composition of the Palaeolithic diet cannot be accurately determined but recent isotopic data from neanderthal and upper Palaeolithic European skeletons support the higher protein dietary intake. Our ancestors ate a higher protein, higher fat, and lower carbohydrate diet.

The sanctioned "healthy diet" is a high carbohydrate, low protein, and low-fat diet. This does not make sense because our species is not adapted to this proportion of macronutrients.

4. Micronutrient composition

A micronutrient is defined as a nutrient needed in small amounts for normal growth and development and these usually refer to dietary components such as vitamins and minerals.

Western diets consist of many refined foods, which, by definition, have many of the micronutrients removed. As well, a large proportion of the soils where crops are grown is mineral depleted; also, artificial fertilizers change the soil pH which affects the mineral content of the crops. All in all, this means that the food grown is minerally deficient. Animals are artificially fed and as such are eating a diet that is un-natural for them and this also alters the level of micronutrients in their bodies. Many crops are picked green and ripen during transport. This reduces the natural ability of fruits and vegetables to develop their optimal vitamin levels. In the end, these depleted fruits and vegetables are kept in cold storage or on supermarket shelves for varying periods of time and what nutrient value they had, is even more depleted. For these reasons, most of the commercial foods we buy are deficient in micronutrients.

Our ancestors ate a fresh diet, unrefined and mostly grown in non-depleted soils. The animals they hunted and ate were free range and ate what animals should normally eat; therefore, the meat of those animals contained an optimal micronutrient content.

5. Acid-base balance

Some foods result in an acid residual after digestion and metabolism, while other foods leave an alkaline residual. Meats are generally acidic, whereas fruits, vegetables and nuts are alkaline. The most acidic producing foods are refined grains and any energy-dense, nutrient poor food. The typical western diet has an overall acidic residual, which in turn, can develop into a low-grade metabolic acidosis which can lead to various diseases such as kidney stones, osteoporosis, hypertension, age-related muscle wasting, and age related chronic renal insufficiency.

Our ancestral diet consisting of meats and fruits and vegetables and nuts (and an absence of grains and other refined foods) had a net alkaline residual, which had a preventative role in the above-mentioned diseases.

6. Sodium-potassium ratio

There is an inversion of the sodium/potassium concentration in the western diet. Our ancestral diet had a higher potassium and a lower sodium ratio. However, due to the use of refined salt (containing mainly sodium and chloride but not any of the other minerals) and the displacement of fruits and vegetables with higher potassium content in favour of grains which have a lower potassium content, the typical western diet is higher in sodium and lower in potassium. This sodium/potassium reversal has contributed to the development of many modern diseases such as hypertension, stroke, kidney stones, osteoporosis, cancers, asthma, insomnia, and tinnitus.

7. Fibre content

The fibre content of a typical American diet is 15 grams per day, which is much lower than the recommended amount of 25-30 grams per day. A diet of refined sugars, dairy products, alcohol, vegetable oils, refined carbohydrates and starchy vegetables is quite low in fibre. Also note that the ancestral diet was high in vegetable fibre, not grain fibre. A low fibre diet has been implicated in conditions such as constipation, varicose veins, haemorrhoids, diverticulosis, hiatus hernia and gastroesophageal reflux. A low fibre diet can also affect our gut microbiota which can influence the development of MetS. Our ancestors ate a diet much higher in fibre, estimated to be around 42.5 grams per day.

The above discussion demonstrates clearly that the modern western diet is deficient in many ways and has changed dramatically from our ancestral diet: the diet we evolved with, the diet that we, as human beings, are genetically and physiologically more adapted to.

This deficiency is due partly to the newly introduced foods we eat but also to the way these foods are grown and processed. The foods most eaten by modern man; cereal grains, dairy and refined sugar are very recent additions to the diet.

These are the foods that cause most of the

problems.

Gut microbiota

MetS and the gut microbiota are connected.

The western diet is low in fibre and protein, but high in "bad" fats and sugar. These, in addition to the stresses and sedentary lifestyle can lead to dyslipidaemia, IR, and inflammation.

The diet, especially low in fibre, the lifestyle, and environmental factors can impact the microbiota, which in turn can influence the development of IR and MetS (Dabke, Hendrick, & Devkota, 2019).

Thomas et al. (2022) wrote *"Unhealthy diets have been shown to induce alterations in the gut microbiota and contribute to the pathogenesis of MetS by altering microbiota composition and disrupting the intestinal barrier, which leads to low-grade systemic inflammation."*

> *"All diseases begin in the gut."*
> **Hippocrates (c460 – c370 BCE)**

There are three types of "food" (and I put "food" in inverted commas for a reason), that humans should not eat, or if they do, it should be only in minimal quantities. They are sugar, grains, and dairy. Just reflect on these "foods" for a while. They represent a very large portion of the western diet, and it is not necessarily healthy.

Considering the above, it comes as no surprise that the level of disease in our society is growing to unprecedented proportions. This, as I said in my introduction, is largely related to our diet. A way of eating we never should have started in the first place. In fact, the introduction of grains into our diet was perhaps *"one of the worst mistakes in the history of the human race"* (Diamond, 1987).

The deadly quartet

The four conditions that I mentioned earlier, i.e. high cholesterol, hypertension, obesity, and diabetes, were lumped together and called the "deadly quartet" by Kaplan in 1989.

In the same year, Reaven and Hoffman showed that hypertensive patients were hyperinsulinaemic when compared to normal controls. They speculated that earlier studies of blood pressure lowering did not improve coronary artery disease rates because the underlying metabolism was not addressed.

The **M**ultiple **R**isk **F**actor **I**ntervention **T**rial otherwise known as MRFIT ("Mister Fit") was sponsored by the US government and cost $115 million. This was a ten-year study of over 12,000 males, aged between 35 and 57 and who were obese, smokers, had poor dietary habits and mild hypertension. Half of the group was given dietary advice and β blockers and/or diuretics to lower the hypertension. The other half was not given anything special and acted as the controls. The results of the trial were surprising. The treated group did achieve a drop in blood pressure, 87% achieved a drop below diastolic 105, and 66% were able to drop below diastolic 90, i.e. to a normal level.

The results seemed to produce a great success. The medication administered can lower elevated diastolic blood pressure, in other words reduce the risk factors, however after ten years, it was found that there was no significant difference in the death rates in the two groups. This result was not expected. In mild-to-moderate hypertension, there seemed to be little benefit from treatment (Multiple Risk Factor Intervention Trial Research Group., 1982).

Further research showed that high insulin levels

are the underlying cause for most of the health problems experienced by the participants in the study. Just reducing the BP does not reduce the insulin levels.

In 1985, a similar study was carried out, and gave similar results. Over 17,000 men and (this time) women with diastolic blood pressure between 90 and 105 were enrolled in this study. Again, they were divided into two groups. The results showed that the treated group had a smaller number of strokes, but overall, the incidence of heart attacks and death was not different, even though the level of blood pressure was reduced in the treated group. However, they did find that rates of heart attacks and death were lower in non-smokers, than in smokers (Medical Research Council Working Party.,1985).

What is going on here? How can we explain this finding? Lowering the level of a temperature gauge in a car does not fix an underlying problem of an overheating engine. You need to find out why the engine is overheating. In the same way, the case of a high BP, lowering the numbers on a reading with medication does not alter the underlying condition that is causing the hypertension.

Manrique, Johnson, and Sowers (2010) highlighted another factor to consider. They showed that diuretics and β blockers can impair insulin sensitivity, in other words aggravate IR. The drugs usually administered do "lower the numbers" but can aggravate the underlying metabolism. Carella et al. (2010) advised that the older β blockers should not be prescribed in MetS.

Risk factors are not diseases.

The four main symptoms of "the deadly quartet" are diabetes, hypertension, hypercholesterolaemia and obesity. As time goes on, other conditions are continually being added to the list: it is no longer just a quartet. Some of these conditions are dangerous, others are simply annoying.

The following conditions are linked to MetS:

1. cancer,
2. fatty liver,
3. reduced age of menarche,
4. increased stature,
5. myopia,
6. skin tags,
7. acanthosis nigricans,
8. polycystic ovary syndrome (PCOS),

9. male vertex balding,
10. gallstones,
11. Alzheimer's disease,
12. acne vulgaris.

The most effective way to treat these varied conditions is to treat the underlying metabolic problem as well as the superficial manifestations. Once the underlying metabolism is addressed, the superficial treatments can be reduced and possibly even stopped.

Why hyperinsulinaemia?

What causes the body to produce more insulin?

The answer is simple: it is due to what we eat and how we live our lives.

This is why I called this book **Death by Civilization**.

To understand how all of this is all related we must now explore the role of insulin.

Insulin

Everybody has heard of insulin. To most, it is the hormone used to treat diabetes. Most think that its only purpose is to reduce blood sugar levels (BSL). Not so. Insulin does a lot more: in fact, reducing the BSL is only a secondary action.

Insulin is a very old molecule; it has been around for millions of years, and it is common to most living things. Even single cell organisms have insulin. One of the actions is to regulate lifespan. When we see that one of the main actions of insulin is to store energy and nutrients, we can see how this fits in. When there is plenty of food around, organisms can live, grow, and reproduce quickly. When there is a scarcity of nutrients, things slow down, and the organism can live longer.

Intermittent fasting, periodic fasting, and especially calorie restriction has been shown to increase lifespan in yeasts, invertebrates, rats, non-human primates, as well as humans (Longo, Di Tano, Mattson, & Guidi, 2021).

Centenarian (people who live to one hundred years or more) studies have shown that these long-lived people have very little in common: specifically, there is no correlation to cholesterol levels, to exercise, to smoking or drinking to whether they are nice or nasty or calm or irritable. However, in one aspect there is a common element: they have relatively low blood sugar levels, low triglycerides and they all have relatively low insulin levels.

Insulin can be regarded as a marker for longevity.

Conversely, IR is a marker for ageing, early death, and disease, especially those diseases that are referred to as the **diseases of civilization**.

The role of insulin is to store energy and nutrients. Our ancestors lived in a harsh environment: food was not necessarily a regular occurrence. When hungry, they couldn't go to the nearest shop or restaurant to get food. It was a matter of finding food or not eating. So, during evolution, a survival mechanism developed, often referred to as the "thrifty gene". Perhaps the term "thrifty genotype" would be better because studies have shown that there is not one gene that does all of this; there are probably many genes working together, thus giving the large variations found.

Basically, the system worked (and works) like this: during times of plenty, when the blood sugar levels were higher, indicating feast times, the body would store this energy in the form of fat, to use during times of famine, as the body "knew" that at some point in time there would be famine conditions. So anytime there was excess energy or nutrients available, the body would store some as glycogen, in the liver and muscles, which have a limited storage capacity, but most would be stored as saturated fat, an almost unlimited storage capacity.

Our hunter-gatherer ancestors developed this ability as a survival mechanism. As civilization developed, food sources became more reliable, so this storage capacity began to work overtime. As humans became more civilised, the diet changed, from the adapted hunter-gatherer diet, high in protein, fat and unrefined vegetables, tubers, nuts, berries, and fruits, (this also includes times when there was no food to eat) to the modern sanctioned concept of the "healthy diet." This concept is one of regularly eating three meals a day consisting of foods high in grains and sugars and low in fat.

The insulin producing pancreatic cells are working overtime to increase the amount of insulin to shunt all this excess energy to fat. This leads to the whole nation becoming fatter and fatter and more and more unhealthy.

What was initially a survival mechanism is now leading to our downfall.

So far, we have seen that insulin stores energy in the form of fat.

What else does it store?

Insulin is an anabolic hormone: it builds protein and muscle. This is borne out by the fact that some body builders are injecting themselves with insulin in addition to supplementing amino acids to build up muscle

(Wolfe, 2000).

Insulin stores magnesium (Mg). Mg is an essential mineral needed for muscle and nerve function as well as being a cofactor for many enzymes. Mg is an intra-cellular mineral: insulin is needed to allow Mg into the cells. The problem here is that if the body becomes insulin resistant, Mg cannot enter the cells, stays in the blood, and is ultimately filtered through the kidneys and lost in the urine; the body becomes Mg deficient.

A low cellular Mg will have many effects, including low energy production.

Mg is also very important in the action and manufacture of insulin. High insulin levels reduce Mg which in turn makes the cells more insulin resistant. Insulin also increases calcium (Ca) excretion, so no matter how much Ca you take, if insulin levels are high, most will go out in the urine, which can lead to osteoporosis.

Muscles tighten up, and if the muscles of the arteries tighten up then the lumen of the artery becomes narrower, i.e. they constrict and therefore, the heart must pump harder to push blood through the narrowed arteries. This leads to higher blood pressure, which is a symptom of MetS.

Insulin also causes sodium retention, which in turn causes water retention and again causes high blood pressure and congestive heart failure, as there is more fluid to pump around the body. At the same time, the heart becomes weaker due to the reduction of energy production.

Insulin is also a strong stimulator of the sympathetic nervous system (SNS) and one of its actions is to constrict the arteries.

Heart attacks are 2-3 times more common after a high carbohydrate meal (and less likely after a high fat meal) due to high insulin levels stimulating the SNS and causing arterial spasm.

High insulin levels cause retention of sodium and water; insulin stimulates the SNS and further constricts the arteries. No wonder this is a prime time for some heart problems.

Insulin influences blood fats. It raises triglyceride levels. Insulin, or should I say IR raises the low-density lipoproteins (LDL) that are thought to have a strong effect on the production of arterial plaque.

I have mentioned IR many times. What does this mean? Basically, the body becomes insensitive, (stops listening) to insulin. The body must release more and more insulin to get the body to respond. Serum insulin levels rise. The beta cells in the pancreas that produce insulin are very robust and can secrete huge amounts of insulin for a long time.

But why does the body stop listening to insulin? The exact mechanism is not known for sure but there are a few factors involved.

Since our ancestors lived in a harsh environment, the main problem was lack of food, and therefore a lack of energy. So, most of the hormonal mechanisms that developed were to keep the BSL up, rather than to reduce it. Hormones such as cortisol, growth hormone, adrenaline and glucagon raise BSL. There is only one hormone that can lower BSL and that is insulin. BSL is reduced because insulin pushes glucose into the muscles. With the modern western diet, high in sugars and refined carbohydrates, insulin is over-stimulated. While the body can still respond to insulin, BSL can drop excessively. This drop in BSL stimulates cortisol. adrenaline is also released which produces nervousness and stimulates the brain to crave more sugar (since there is a low sugar state). This craving makes people eat more sugar, which produces an insulin release which again can drop the BSL, and the process is repeated. This ongoing rise and fall in the BSL disturbs the body; and don't forget, all this time cortisol is also being secreted as the body is being stressed. Cortisol does add to the development of diabetes.

Every time there is a rise in BSL, insulin is secreted. Every time the body is exposed to this excess surge of insulin, the cells become more resistant. Insulin does reduce the BSL. So, every time there is a surge of insulin, BSL can drop, possibly even too low which can lead to hypoglycaemia (low blood sugar). This produces symptoms of fast heart rate, dizziness, sweating, fainting, hunger, anxiety, and confusion. Note that there are many people who feel sleepy and fuzzy headed after a high carbohydrate meal (reactive hypoglycaemia). This is due to the excess drop in the BSL. While the body is still partially responsive to insulin, BSL drops too low in response to the high insulin surge. The body does not like these repeated drops in BSL, so to protect itself, the body starts to switch off the insulin receptors, slowly increasing the IR. The BSL needs to be kept at a specified level, not too low or too high. A high carbohydrate meal stimulates the pancreas to release insulin which drops the BSL. In the short term, this possibly leads to little harm but in the long term, may lead to IR.

The cells become more resistant, so the body secretes more insulin (hyperinsulinaemia) to try to keep the BSL in the normal range. This process continues and the BSL may remain stable even as the insulin levels progressively get higher. Eventually, however, the body becomes so resistant that the insulin loses any effect and the BSL rises above the pre-set level. This is the beginning of type 2 diabetes (T2D), another symptom of MetS.

Insulin is a two-edged sword. We need insulin to maintain life, but too much insulin can cause problems. The condition of type 1 diabetes (T1D) is where there is no insulin production. Treatment involves administering insulin injections.

What if too much insulin is given?

Intensive T1D treatment

A high insulin level can lead to MetS. A treatment method commonly used for T1D is "intensive insulin treatment", which is a treatment method involving the use of multiple doses of insulin, and regular BSL monitoring to keep the BSL in a "tight range." This may reduce the T1D complications but, if overdone, can be associated with excess weight gain, central obesity, and dyslipidaemia. This, in turn, can lead to IR, hypertension, and more extensive atherosclerosis (Purnell, Zinman, Brunzell, DCCT/EDIC Research Group, 2013).

This sounds a lot like MetS.

We can consider this a form of iatrogenic (doctor

caused) hyperinsulinaemia, leading to iatrogenic MetS.

An essential mineral for maintaining the BSL is chromium (Cr). Cr is needed for the proper function of the insulin receptors. High sugar, carbohydrate diets tend to push Cr out through the urine, so the body becomes Cr depleted. This adds to IR. Therefore, one of the main treatments needed to restore insulin receptor function is Cr supplementation.

Why all this talk about sugar and carbohydrates?

Isn't it obvious?

The western diet is excessively high in sugar and carbohydrates, especially refined carbohydrates: white sugar, HFCS, white bread, white noodles, cereals, and other ultra-processed foods.

Different tissues become resistant at different rates. Some cells become resistant very easily, others become resistant very slowly; some hardly become resistant at all.

The liver is the first that can become resistant and as we know, the liver is possibly one of the most metabolically active organs of the body. IR will interfere with liver function.

The muscles are next to become resistant. If the

muscles are resistant, they cannot absorb the sugar, and so become weak and tired, which also makes it more difficult for BSL to be reduced.

The third tissue that becomes resistant is the fat cells. While the fat cells are not (yet) resistant, more and more sugar, under the influence of insulin, is converted to fat and stored. This leads to obesity, another symptom of MetS.

One tissue that hardly becomes resistant is the endothelium, the lining of the arteries. So, this high level of insulin continues to influence the lining of the arteries. Insulin is an anabolic hormone; it stimulates proliferation and cell division. Since the endothelium is very resistant to becoming insulin resistant, the high insulin levels cause the artery lining to grow, thicken and to develop plaques.

Insulin also influences blood clotting, increasing platelet adhesiveness. Insulin also influences converting macrophages to foam cells … and here we have it … the circle is complete! High sugar, carbohydrate diet causes insulin release which causes atherosclerosis and increased blood clotting which leads to cardiovascular disease. Cardiovascular disease is a symptom of MetS.

The vicious cycle continues, becoming an ever-worsening situation. The body becomes increasingly resistant as it secretes more and more insulin. Eventually, the high level of insulin produces all the damage that we have already discussed.

A good question to ask is "When does insulin sensitivity start?"

Does it start in early adulthood? "No"

Does it start in childhood? "No"

Does it start in infancy? "No"

It starts even before that.

What?!!!

Establishment of insulin sensitivity begins as soon as sperm meets egg. Now here comes the frightening bit. If sperm meets egg in a high insulin environment, that embryo becomes more prone to develop hyperinsulinaemia and IR (Plagemann, Harder, Kohlhoff, Rohde, & Dörner, 1997; Weiss et al., 2000).

A good question to ask is *"What is a high insulin environment?"* A pregnant mother with gestational diabetes mellitus (GDM) would fit this description. It gets worse. An obese mother without GDM would also fit this description, as obesity can indicate hyperinsulinaemia.

Boney, Verma, Tucker, and Vohr (2005) demonstrated that an obese mother, with or without GDM, would conceive and produce an already extra insulin sensitive child. The child would be more likely to become IR and develop obesity, hypertension, and diabetes i.e. MetS in the future.

It is frightening that we see so many obese pregnant women around.

An article by Elissa Doherty (2007) in Adelaide's *Sunday Mail* highlights the concern about this. *"Overweight pregnant women are becoming too big for beds at the Woman's and Children's Hospital as weight problems in mothers-to-be hit record levels."*

"Top SA doctors have warned oversized pregnant women are increasingly putting at risk not only their lives and health, but their children's."

"The trend is also setting children on the path to obesity from the womb..."

What is even more frightening is, if that foetus is a female, then the developing eggs in that foetus' ovaries are already more insulin sensitive, therefore they become insulin resistant more easily, so subsequent generations may be affected.

This whole situation is becoming increasingly

worse, hence the comments in my introduction that any positive change will take not years but generations.

Leptin

I think it is an appropriate time to introduce leptin. Leptin (from the Greek *leptos*, meaning thin) is a hormone secreted by fat cells. The fat cells are not an inert fat storage system but a part of the complicated system that regulates energy and storage. Here, in effect, the fat cells are acting as an endocrine organ. Leptin is the hormone that feeds back to the brain information on the level of stored fat/energy. The more fat stored, the more leptin is released. Leptin levels are monitored by the brain, and this has the effect of reducing appetite and increasing metabolism. If there is less fat storage, then there is less leptin, and this has the effect of increasing appetite and reducing metabolism.

Leptin gives the brain an index of energy storage.

When leptin was first discovered, there was great excitement. This could be a way to deal with the obesity problem: drug companies had dollar ign in their eye$!

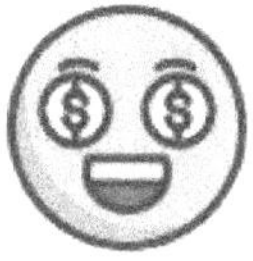

Some experiments were done on mice, and overweight mice lost weight with leptin injections, but this was *only* in cases where there was a leptin deficiency. (No leptin: the brain thinks the storage is low, so the mouse eats and eats and eats.) There are some very rare, usually hereditary, cases amongst humans where there is leptin deficiency. Leptin injections do help these rare cases. However, obese people do not have a leptin deficiency. Leptin levels are found to be high. This should give the signal to the brain to reduce appetite, but this is not occurring.

Why?

What is happening is a leptin resistance, analogous to IR: the fat cells are secreting lots of leptin, but the brain is not listening. The brain interprets this as a low leptin state and appetite is not reduced. Excess hunger leads to continuous eating. Research on leptin is still in the very early stages and a lot is not known, so watch this space.

What is known is that there is some interaction between insulin and leptin. These two hormones have some opposing actions such as lipogenesis and fatty acid oxidation, but in other aspects they work together. Leptin is known to inhibit insulin secretion and biosynthesis.

Insulin and leptin work together to control metabolism. Insulin tends to work mainly at the individual cell level while leptin works more on the whole of the body generally via the SNS, although there is some evidence for some direct effect on the muscle and fat cells.

Leptin also has connections to the immune system, the reproductive system and, in fact, to almost every other system. As far as reproduction goes, low energy stores produce low levels of leptin, which interferes with the ability to menstruate, and to get pregnant. When you think about it, it does make perfect sense. Imagine our Palaeolithic ancestor during a time of famine; the stored fat energy is used up. This is possibly the worst time to get pregnant, not just for the mother but also the child. Nature has developed a fail-safe device. The low leptin levels tell the brain there is very little storage, so this low leptin level switches off the reproductive cycle.

The whole leptin story is very complex and is not yet fully understood.

While leptin is working properly, as soon as the fat storage increases, the cells release leptin, and this tells the brain to reduce appetite. When leptin is low, the brain gets the message to increase appetite but, in this complicated world, this feedback loop breaks down. The exact reason or reasons are not known for sure. It could be due to the diet, perhaps the high carbohydrate diet producing IR (as discussed before) which, in turn, can lead to leptin resistance.

Leptin must enter the brain through the blood brain barrier (BBB) to have its effects on the SNS signalling system. Leptin must be transported through the BBB. Banks et al. (2004) showed that triglycerides inhibit leptin transport through the BBB.

Note that a high sugar diet and IR leads to high serum triglycerides.

Not all parts of the brain become equally resistant; some parts of the brain get a reduced message, while other parts still get the full message. The appetite centre seems to become resistant early on, so it does not get the message to curb hunger. The person continues to eat excessively and gain weight. The leptin levels rise, yet the appetite centre is still not getting the message to stop. On the other hand, the control centre of the SNS is not as resistant and gets the full message of the high leptin levels, leading to over stimulation of the SNS, which can lead to diabetes, elevated BP, increased blood coagulation, heart disease and increased inflammation.

The way to fix leptin resistance is firstly to deal with the IR problem. This is achieved by reducing carbohydrates and sugars in the diet, reducing snacking, and generally eating less. Fasting for short periods, as well as to supplement nutrients such as chromium (Cr) and omega 3 fish oils can also help. One specific way to reduce leptin is to exercise, which can help IR as well. Sleep is also an important issue. Lack of sleep can increase leptin secretion. Conversely, more sleep can reduce it.

Some specific nutrients have been shown to affect leptin physiology. Gangloff et al. (2020) demonstrated that vitamin D is a potent leptin secretion inhibitor.

This is important because the level of vitamin D in the community is generally low. How can this be so? We, in Australia, live in a very sunny climate. Vitamin D deficiency is possibly due to the “Slip, Slop, Slap” campaign. While it may be good to prevent skin cancer, the campaign has become too efficient; the pendulum has swung too far the other way. People are now scared, even paranoid, to go out in the sun: you could say they have had the “living daylights scared out of them”! Sensible sunning is required, not sunburn; 15-20 minutes in full, midday sun will give adequate vitamin D. If for some reason, the person cannot get into the sun, then vitamin D3 supplements can be given. The evidence is that vitamin D3 is a better supplement than vitamin D2

(Balachandar, Pullakhandam, Kulkarni, & Sachdev, 2021).

Another nutrient that has been shown to reduce leptin resistance is conjugated linoleic acid (CLA) (Mohammadi-Sartang, Sohrabi, Esmaeilinezhad, Aqaeinezhad, & Jalilpiran, 2018).

CLA is a mixture of positional and geometric isomers of linoleic acid. CLA can be found in milk, cheese, butter, and yoghurt – (note that dairy sources may have negative effects, especially if there is dairy allergy or intolerance.) Eggs, and meat, from free range, grass fed, (not grain fed, feedlot) animals also contain CLA. A particular good source in Australia is kangaroo and wallaby meat.

The western diet is terrible.

Humans were not designed to eat such a diet. It is too high in refined carbohydrates, sugars, and excess bad fats.

Excess carbohydrates and sugars stimulate the pancreas to release insulin. This is normal, that is what the system was designed to do. However, there is always a "however", this mechanism developed on a diet that was very low in refined carbohydrates and sugar.

Our species evolved in the Palaeolithic era when

humans were hunter-gatherers; our genes and our physiology are still Palaeolithic. Our genes have not changed, yet our diet has.

The Palaeolithic diet was varied, depending on season, and on location. It was also based on availability. Our Palaeolithic ancestors could not nip into the local deli or pizza restaurant when hungry. They had to hunt and gather. This meant they had to exercise to get their food. There were times when the hunt failed and there was no food. There were times when our Palaeolithic ancestors did not eat. To survive those harsh times, a mechanism developed where energy was stored in the form of fat during times of plenty to enable survival during the lean times. Of course, now, there is continuous plenty, there are no lean times, and the diet is much different. This mechanism, the "thrifty gene", is working overtime.

What was a mechanism designed to assist us in our survival, is now harming us.

The "thrifty gene" hypothesis has been debated for many years since Neel proposed it in 1996. There have been many criticisms of this hypothesis. However, Hales and Barker (2001) write that many studies have confirmed the initial evidence although the strength of the evidence does vary with the different studies. One thing is clear, and that is its relationship to IR at all ages studied. Venniyoor (2020) agreed that the "thrifty gene" did help the organism to survive famine by improving energy efficiency and storing excess energy as fat and this gene has become detrimental because of the modern obesogenic environment. He also proposed that it is the phosphatase and tensin homolog (PTEN) gene that is calibrated in utero by methylation to "fix" this metabolic capacity.

The Palaeolithic diet has been estimated to be much higher in protein and fat, especially in omega 3 fatty acids, high in vegetables, fruits, and nuts, very low in refined carbohydrates and to contain virtually zero sugar.

The twenty-first century diet is high in sugars, refined carbohydrates, vegetable oils, rancid and trans fatty acids, and low in fat and protein. The few vegetables we do eat are very low in vitamins and minerals.

Cordain et al. (2005) wrote; *"Although dairy products, cereals, refined sugars, refined vegetable oils and alcohol make up 72.1% of the total daily energy consumed by all people in the United States, these types of foods would have contributed little or none of the energy in the typical preagriculture hominin diet."*

Dairy, cereals, refined sugar, refined vegetable oil

are very new additions to the human diet. We have not (yet) adapted to such a diet. Perhaps in another 10,000 to 20,000 years we may, if we don't become extinct first.

Considering what has been discussed up until this point, you may be thinking that only the diet is causing this abnormal metabolism.

Unfortunately, not so.

A lack of exercise is another issue.

"The two basic forces spreading this malady (i.e. MetS) *are the increase in consumption of high calorie-low fiber fast food and the decrease in physical activity due to mechanized transportations and sedentary form of leisure time activities"*
(Saklayen, 2018).

There are other contributions.

Our ancestors not only ate differently but their lifestyle was different. They were more active, slept more, were out in the sun more and were less stressed. These factors are important in the development of MetS.

Stress has been shown to be a cause of MetS: and

if you haven't noticed, there is a lot of stress in today's modern society.

Another factor, which is closely related to stress, is sleep, or should I say, lack of. Our ancestors developed a circadian rhythm with the sun. They woke up with the sun and went to sleep when the sun went down and became dark.

Sleep

Over many thousands of years, over countless generations, humanity has used the sun as a giant clock and developed a hard-wired biological rhythm based on light and dark periods. Our ancestors woke up when the sun came up and went to sleep when the sun went down and became dark. Of course, this does depend on where you live. Higher latitudes had excess long or short hours of light depending on the season.

They had campfires and torches and oil lamps that gave off only a low intensity lighting, but generally they went to sleep as soon as darkness fell. With the invention of improved artificial lighting, then later, electricity, another unnatural life-style change occurred which goes against the grain of thousands of years of evolution. The modern population is staying up later and later; and consequently, sleeping much less.

In the past the nights were dark; now, night can be as bright as day. Shops and factories are working 24 hours a day. Shift work is having a negative effect on the health of workers.

Everyone needs a good night's sleep … but how much is that? In the past the usual amount of sleep was much more than today because of the cycle of the sun. People are sleeping less (Sheehan, Frochen, Walsemann, & Ailshire, 2019).

Owen et al. (2014) have shown that lack of sleep has consequences, including depression, increased risk of obesity, and higher rates of drowsy driving accidents.

Taheri, Lin, Austin, Young, and Mignot (2004) showed that sleep deprivation can alter levels of leptin and ghrelin, two hormones that cause increase in hunger and appetite which can lead to increased body weight. Ghrelin, produced by the stomach, is a hormone that stimulates appetite.

Sleep deprivation has been shown to cause MetS. Studies, as discussed below, have shown that people who sleep less have more hypertension, more obesity, more diabetes, and more cancer, which is basically MetS.

Che et al. (2021) showed a U-shaped relationship

between sleep duration and MetS. Too short or too long a sleep is associated with MetS. In this study, short sleep was defined as less than six hours of sleep, while too long sleep was defined as greater than eight hours sleep. There must be a "Goldilocks's zone"; not too much, not too little, just the right amount.

Another issue is insomnia: difficulty getting to sleep or staying asleep. This condition is very common. Roth (2007) estimates that at least 30% of the population have some degree of insomnia. Insomnia can be related to pain, anxiety, drugs, alcohol, sleep apnoea, and age. About 40% of those with insomnia have some form of comorbid psychiatric conditions.

The basis of sleep is the hormone melatonin. Light entering the eye is signalled to the pineal gland, the part of the brain that controls and produces the sleep hormone, melatonin. This has a regulating effect on the light/dark cycle.

Light suppresses the production of this hormone, so the more light entering the eye, the less melatonin produced, which influences other hormones including prolactin, glucocorticoids, serotonin, ACTH, and cortisol.

Melatonin can regulate, and therefore alter, metabolism, immune function, and endocrine balance, which include IR, the basic underlying cause of MetS. Melatonin has been shown by Li and Xu (2021) to reduce insulin levels and improve insulin sensitivity.

Excess light and lack of sleep, both of which lead to reduced melatonin levels, are a cause of MetS.

As the population is sleeping less and less, the metabolism is changing, leading to an epidemic of obesity, diabetes, hypertension, and cancer. That is, MetS.

The time to eat has also changed. In medieval times and even perhaps earlier, the main meal was in the middle of the day, i.e. during daylight hours. This makes sense, as it is difficult preparing food in the dark. The rich started the trend to eat main meals at night because they could afford to have artificial lighting.

For most of us today, the main meal is at night.

The adage *"eat breakfast like a king, lunch like a prince, and dinner like a pauper"* has many advocates but how true is this? The research is contradictory.

I remember reading an article written by a Sumo wrestler who wrote that the way to put on weight, which is important for Sumo wrestlers, is to fast all day, then have a big meal at night and go to sleep. This will put on weight. From this we would assume that if you want to lose weight, or at least not put on more weight, then you should do the opposite.

Does eating the last thing at night cause obesity? Some seem to think so, although it may relate to a person's chronotype i.e. whether they are a "morning person" or a "night person" (Xiao, Garaulet, & Scheer, 2019).

Davis, Rogers, Coates, Leung, and Bonham (2022) concluded that, *"The literature summarised in this review highlights emerging evidence that the timing of food intake can impact weight gain and increased adiposity, with night and later meal timings negatively impacting weight regulation favouring the development of obesity over time."*

Also note,

- Being up later and later will cause an increase in snacking (which generally is high sugar and refined carbohydrate) and this causes weight gain. (Note that these snacks are extra food intake) and
- Lack of, or reduced sleep, can cause weight gain because of the relationship between sleep and MetS.

Exercise

Our ancestors were very active, yet today's population is very inactive. Exercise is an important lifestyle factor in the treatment and prevention of MetS.

Hawley (2004) showed that regular exercise improves IR, which is the underlying problem in MetS. Exercise can help to lose weight, to improve blood pressure, and to improve BSL.

By exercise, I do not necessarily mean you have to go to the gym and lift weights (unless you particularly want to), the important thing is to keep active. Walking is possibly the best exercise. Walk instead of using the car, especially if you only need to go a short distance. Use the stairs instead of the lift. Stop one or two bus stops earlier and walk the rest.

There is another advantage of walking - it will get you outdoors and into the sunshine.

Sunshine and vitamin D

Sunshine is important; it is our main source of vitamin D. Why is this important? A deficiency of vitamin D is another cause of MetS. Those with MetS have been found to have lower levels of vitamin D

(Melguizo-Rodríguez et al., 2021).

Vitamin D has been shown to have a positive correlation with insulin sensitivity and a negative correlation with pancreatic beta cell function. In other words, vitamin D deficiency can cause increased IR and have an adverse effect on the pancreatic cells that produce insulin (Chiu, Chu, Go, & Saad, 2004).

Supplementing vitamin D can improve the situation.

Those with low vitamin D levels are more predisposed to developing MetS. When treating anyone with MetS, vitamin D levels should be checked and, if needed, supplemented. Vitamin D has a direct relationship with all the facets of MetS: i.e. diabetes, obesity, hypertension, cholesterol, and cancer. Vitamin D can be supplemented in the form of vitamin D3 and/or by encouraging more sunshine exposure.

I advise my patients to get sun exposure, not sunburn.

Treat the underlying metabolism.

Pesticides and other chemicals

Another cause of MetS is the myriads of chemicals released into the environment, which include bisphenol A (BPA), per- and polyfluoroalkyl substances (PFASs), phthalates, polycyclic aromatic hydrocarbons (PAHs), pesticides and heavy metals, such as cadmium (Cd), arsenic (As), lead (Pb), and mercury (Hg).

Pesticides may produce a short-term benefit with increased crop yields, however, as Arab and Mostafalou (2023) showed *"There are also some evidences on the link of exposure to pesticides with higher incidence of metabolic diseases associated with insulin resistance like diabetes, obesity, metabolic syndrome, hypertension, polycystic ovary syndrome and chronic kidney diseases."*

Lamat et al. (2022) came to the same conclusion.

De Long and Holloway (2017) took it one step further and showed that chemicals in general, not just pesticides can predispose to MetS, especially if exposure was at an early age. *"This narrative review explores the evidence linking early-life exposure to a suite of chemicals that are common contaminants associated with food production (pesticides; imidacloprid, chlorpyrifos, and glyphosate) and processing (acrylamide), in addition to chemicals ubiquitously found in our household goods (brominated flame retardants) and drinking water (heavy metals) and changes in key pathways important for the development of MetS and obesity."*

See also Haverinen, Fernandez, Mustieles, and Tolonen (2021).

Glyphosate is the most common herbicide used in the world. Eskenazi et al. (2023) showed that glyphosate exposure between ages five and eighteen were associated with increased rates of liver damage (elevated liver transaminases) and MetS. They also showed that prenatal and childhood exposure from birth to age five was associated with MetS by age eighteen.

Other pollutants are heavy metals. Xu et al. (2021) showed heavy metal exposure was positively associated with MetS.

As part of the treatment of MetS, not only should the diet be changed to organic foods, and avoiding chemicals, pesticides, and herbicides as much as possible, but other life-style factors need to be addressed. This must include more sleep, more exercise, more vitamin D, and less stress (easier said than done). Avoiding heavy metals should also be considered but this may be hard to do. We cannot live in a bubble.

Dutch winter famine

The Dutch famine of 1944 -1945 occurred towards the end of World War 2 (WW2), in the German occupied Netherlands. This was caused by a combination of a harsh winter, poor crops, four years of war and a German blockade of food shipments. Thousands died and millions were affected. The reason the Dutch winter famine is mentioned is because there is a cohort of people being studied who were not yet born but their mothers were pregnant during the famine. This cohort has been studied extensively. What is found is that the people who were *in utero* during the famine were found to have a high incidence of MetS as well as other issues, compared to those born before or after the famine.

Kyle and Pichard (2016) comment that *"Exposure to famine during gestation resulted in increases in impaired glucose tolerance, obesity, coronary heart disease, atherogenic lipid profile, hypertension, microalbuminuria, schizophrenia, antisocial personality and affective disorders."*

Loke (2014) showed that foetuses exposed to famine during mid to late gestation developed reduced glucose tolerance with increased IR. Foetuses exposed to famine in early gestation developed a more atherogenic profile, obesity, and a higher risk of coronary heart disease.

Loke (2014) also discussed the issue of the Chinese famine from 1959 to 1961. Adults who were exposed to famine during their foetal life had a higher risk of developing MetS.

What could have caused this?

The answer is probably epigenetics. Epigenetics is where the environment can alter gene expression. The actual DNA does not change but various genes can be switched on or off in response to the environment. The switched on/switched off genes can be passed on to the next few generations. This gene expression alteration is based on methylation (Tobi et al., 2009).

It seems that both over-eating, and famine can affect the developing foetus and can predispose the child in later life to develop MetS. We are killing ourselves by our diet, lifestyle, as well as the pollution. This is why I call this book **Death by Civilization**.

A Typical Scenario

How many times have you seen patients who are apparently healthy and on routine examination have been found to be hypertensive. There more than likely is a family history of hypertension (or any combination of diabetes, obesity or hypercholesterolaemia, i.e. MetS).

Routine tests are done and are found to be normal. An anti-hypertensive drug is commenced. Over the next few years there is gradual weight gain, especially around the abdomen. Later, high cholesterol is discovered and a cholesterol lowering drug is introduced. As even more time passes, diabetes develops, and they are put on an anti-diabetic drug. The situation would be worsened if the anti-hypertensive drug was a beta blocker and/or a diuretic. This is a typical history of the slow progressive development of MetS. It does not need to come all at once, nor necessarily in the order as described but, in the end, you have a fat, hypertensive, diabetic with elevated cholesterol on multiple medications.

If, right at the beginning, a serum insulin estimation was performed and (more than likely) the patient was found to be hyperinsulinaemic, and if an appropriate lifestyle changes, diet, and supplements had been commenced, then the progression to full MetS may not have occurred. Wouldn't this be cheaper and better for the person in the long run?

OBESITY

"It is very injurious to health to take in more food than the constitution will bear, when, at the same time one uses no exercise to carry off this excess."
Hippocrates (c460-c370 BCE)

The population is getting fatter; it is impossible not to notice this.

But why?

There is an increasing number of obese people. From 2014-2015 the rate of overweight and obesity in those over 18 increased from 63.4% to 67%. In 2017-2018, 67% of Australians over 18 were classed as overweight (35.6%) or obese (31.1%). In 2017-2018 the proportion of overweight and obese men (74.5%) was greater than women (59.7%).

(https://www.abs.gov.au › statistics › health › health-conditions-and-risks › overweight-and-obesity › latest release - Accessed 12 August 2023)

In 2017–18, 25% of Australian children and adolescents aged 2–17 were overweight or obese. Of these, 8.2% were classed as obese.

(https://www.aihw.gov.au › reports › overweight-obesity ›overweight-obesity-australian-children-adolesents/summary - Accessed 12 August 2023)

In the 10 March 2007 edition of the Adelaide Advertiser, an article "*Jumbo ambulance for obese patients" by* journalist Jill Pengelley highlighted the extent of the problem of obesity for the Australian healthcare system. Standard size ambulances cannot cater for the obese. When an ambulance is called for, the weight of the patient will be requested so they can dispatch an appropriately sized ambulance. Even the hospitals need special beds for the obese. Standard beds are not big enough. This is the case with operating room tables as well.

Mortuaries are also having difficulty dealing with obese bodies. Special reinforced equipment is needed. Autopsies have been known to have been done on the floor as lifting the bodies onto the table was next to impossible (Byard, 2012).

Babies are not exempt. Trifiletti et al. (2006) report

that baby capsules need to be made increasingly bigger because more and more babies cannot fit safely into the standard sized safety capsule.

A fast-food chain had to change the fixed tables and chairs. The seating and table had to be moved further apart because people couldn't fit in. To be more flexible, some restaurants are now un-bolting the tables and chairs so that they can be moved. There was even a lawsuit where an obese man sued a burger chain restaurant because the chairs were too small.

Why, relatively suddenly, have a larger and larger proportion of the population become obese?

Obesity is dangerous and can lead to long term ill health and early death: some caused by the obesity itself, though most is caused by the underlying metabolism that I have written about so far. Many of the health problems are associated with obesity, this does not necessarily mean they are "caused" by obesity.

Angelidi, Belanger, Kokkinos, Koliaki, and Mantzoros (2022) estimate that worldwide, the yearly deaths caused by a high body mass index (BMI) i.e. overweight and obesity, to be over four million.

That is a lot of people.

The difficulty is separating deaths from obesity

per se and deaths of obese individuals with associated illnesses. Many of these conditions are associated because the same underlying condition is the cause. Conditions such as cancer, diabetes, hypertension, hypercholesterolaemia, and heart disease are all symptoms of MetS. This leads back to my basic premise: it is not necessarily the superficial manifestations that are the problem but the underlying metabolism.

Obesity is also associated with many varied conditions, including sleep apnoea, osteoarthritis, gout, fertility problems, menstrual problems, and gallbladder disease. Again, these may also be related to the underlying metabolism.

From a purely mechanical point of view, lugging around kilograms of excess weight can affect the heart, the back, the joints, especially the lower limbs, the lungs, as gross obesity makes breathing difficult. Also, obese people tend to get tired easily and therefore do not exercise as much, which can compound the problem: it becomes a vicious cycle.

Obese people have difficulty conceiving. It is well known that obese women have menstrual irregularities, have more difficulty conceiving and are more likely to miscarry (Broughton & Moley, 2017).

If an obese woman does conceive and produces a

baby, the baby has a greater chance of being obese, or becoming obese later in life. They will also, more than likely, produce a next generation of obese adults, which will continue the vicious cycle.

There is also a degree of biased selection. As a general observation, thin healthy active men usually pair off with thin healthy active women and generally produce thin healthy babies.

Again, as a general observation, obese men tend to pair off with obese women and produce babies that are more likely to become obese, so the trend perpetuates.

The incidence of polycystic ovarian syndrome (PCOS) is relatively high amongst the obese and this can be related to hyperinsulinaemia and therefore MetS.

Palmer, Bakos, Fullston, and Lane (2012) demonstrated that fertility problems also occur in obese males. The researchers have shown that obese males have reduced sperm quantity and quality. The researchers noted that male obesity *"... also impairs offspring metabolic and reproductive health suggesting that paternal health cues are transmitted to the next generation ..."*

This may be due to epigenetics.

As I have already noted, the new species of human,

Homo obesissimus, is very unhealthy and relatively infertile. This is reflected in the increasing incidence of those needing assisted fertility treatments.

As a larger and larger proportion of people are mutating to this species, it is only a matter of time before reproduction cannot occur and extinction becomes a possibility.

There have been programmes on the television about the grossly obese in the USA. These people weigh in excess of 200 kilograms and are virtually confined to bed. There are even special nursing homes in the USA (where else??!!), especially designed for the grossly obese! In most cases these people are their own worst enemy. They can eat themselves to death.

There are also many psychological issues involved with obesity.

Although obesity is common, thinner, healthier individuals often look down on the obese, and this produces many psychological issues, such as depression and social isolation. This is now called “fat shaming”. Many are bullied and discriminated against: in the school yard, and in the workplace. The most ironic aspect is that the obese probably outnumber the non-obese at this present point in history.

Even though the majority of the population is

obese or overweight, the ideal, as portrayed by the media, TV, Hollywood, Bollywood, the magazines, the beauty pageants, Miss World, Miss Universe, etc. all emphasize the thin body. There is this dichotomy with what the "ideal body" is and what most of the population are. For the majority, the attainment of these "ideal" body figures is totally unrealistic. Many have body image problems. No wonder there is so much depression and dissatisfaction in the community.

To counter this, the use of positive imaging is being used to advocate that obese bodies are normal, beautiful, and should be admired. Obese women have appeared on the cover of various magazines to try to promote acceptance of the obese body as the "body beautiful". However, this has been criticized saying accepting obesity is a formula for additional negative health issues.

There have been popular TV programmes such as *"Extreme Makeover"* where you too can have the perfect body with plastic surgery, liposuction, etc. Unfortunately, this is all cosmetic/superficial: the underlying metabolism is not addressed.

That other programme *"The Biggest Loser"* does emphasize diet, exercise, and lifestyle more, which is a much better approach.

Even gastric surgery, such as the lap band, is superficial. You may lose weight, but the underlying metabolism may not necessarily change. This can only occur with a change in diet and lifestyle.

Causes of obesity

MetS is not the only cause of obesity, although it is probably the most common.

Other causes include,

- endocrine disease such as Cushing's disease, hypothyroidism,
- medications such as steroids, antipsychotics,
- genetics,
- hormonal problems,
- psychological.

Obviously, the cause of obesity needs to be explored. Is it related to MetS or are there hormonal, endocrine, genetic, or other reasons? These need to be investigated, diagnosed, and treated appropriately.

However, since the most common cause of obesity

is MetS, obesity should be considered as a symptom of the abnormal underlying metabolism; just like diabetes, hypertension, and high cholesterol, which are also only superficial manifestations.

Obesity is a symptom of modern western society and lifestyle.

A British government think-tank released a report in October 2007: *"... the technological revolution of the 20th century has led to weight gain becoming unavoidable for the majority of the population, because <u>our bodies and biological make-up are out of step with our surroundings.</u>"* (Emphasis the author)

A major cause of obesity is the abnormal underlying metabolism caused by a highly refined, carbohydrate rich diet. A diet that has never been experienced by humanity till only relatively recently. So, diet is a very important issue.

If we look at what westerners are eating, it is not hard to see why the population is increasing in obesity. The diet is loaded with sugars and carbohydrates, and the food portions are large and growing.

Who can forget that documentary film *"Super-size me"*? This was an Academy Award nominated documentary film in 2004 by Morgan Spurlock.

This documentary followed him eating only from a well-known fast-food chain for 30 days and exercising less than he usually did. During this time, he put on 11 kilograms, developed depression, lethargy, and headaches, which, not surprisingly, were relieved by eating the fast food. He developed a lack of energy and a reduced sex drive. By day 20 he developed heart palpitations, and his doctors informed him that his liver is being affected. He just managed to finish the 30 days.

It took Morgan Spurlock five months to lose nine kilograms and another nine months to lose the remaining kilograms he put on during the experiment.

Of course, this "experiment" can be criticized (and the fast-food company involved did so) but the point is clear. Eat "junk food", high in calories and sugars and fat and you will get sick. Many people eat these types of food all the time. No wonder we are a sick, unhealthy society.

Our ancestors did *not* have a regular dietary intake, and this was because of the nature of hunting and gathering. There is never a guarantee that food will be supplied on demand. There was always the possibility that the hunt would fail, or no food would be found to be gathered. This being the case, nature had to do something; otherwise, the species would have become extinct through starvation.

A back-up, fail-safe mechanism had to develop to save the species from starving. It goes without saying that our Palaeolithic ancestors could not ring for a dial-a-pizza or rush off to the local supermarket to buy food. Uber eats had not yet been invented!

During times of plenty, excess energy was converted to fat to be used in times of famine. The body "knew" that at some stage there would be famine conditions. Fat is the best form of storing energy as it is calorie rich. This is where the hormone insulin comes into play. We have already explored how insulin contributes to obesity: it is the main energy storage hormone; it converts any excess calories to fat.

The problem today is that we live in times of continual plenty. This survival mechanism designed to store fat during times of plenty is now working full time. Everything we eat, in excess of our needs, is being converted to fat. At the same time, our culture and lifestyle are changing. This is related to the other half of the equation.

One common explanation is that our calorie intake exceeds our calorie output. So, all we must do is eat less and exercise more. This is a very simplistic theory. This has been referred to as the "bucket theory". That is, food/calories being poured into a bucket and exercise takes it out. Any excess will overflow and result in obesity.

The idea that food equals calories (or kilojoules) is not strictly correct. Fat contains more calories than other foods, so this is where the low-fat idea started. We have been browbeaten into believing that we should eat low fat. In the past, advertisements on TV promoted a chain of fast foods that *"contain 6 grams of fat or less"*. A great number of products on the shelves of the supermarket are labelled "low fat" and a very important question to ask is: "If the fat is removed, what is put in its place to make it palatable?" The answer is sugar. So, we are eating less fat, but more sugar.

Is this a con? Yes, I believe it is. The premise that we should eat low fat is politically correct but that does not mean it is true.

Look back at the history of mankind. Fat has been a part of the diet for centuries, so why is it only now that fat has suddenly become a problem? We are, in fact, eating less fat; yet are becoming fatter.

It may sound contradictory but eating fat does not make us fat. In fact, eating more fat can help us lose fat.

Experiments by Kekwick and Pawan in 1956 showed that obese patients lost the most weight on a high fat, low carbohydrate diet. Obese patients lost the least weight on a high carbohydrate, low fat diet. Going back to the calorie counting con, Kekwick and Pawan showed that on a calorie-controlled diet, where most of the calories came from fat, weight was lost, but on a diet with the same number of calories, where the calories were from carbohydrates, weight was gained.

Calories from fat are dealt with differently by the body than calories from carbohydrates.

This is where the bucket theory fails.

Today it is politically incorrect to talk about a high fat/protein diet. The mainstream medicine and media have made the pronouncement that a low fat, high carbohydrate diet is the officially sanctioned diet and that is it. The food police are out there telling us to eat high carb and low fat.

Misinformation

We are being misled, mis-informed.

We are told that low fat is good. The TV, the magazines all advertise low fat, high carb foods. The specially designed “low fat” foods are higher in sugar, which in the end, cause more weight gain.

We are mis-led in other ways too.

For example, fruit juices. They are touted as "healthy", so many parents are feeding their children this "healthy" drink, believing it is the right thing to do. However, the amount of sugar in fruit juice is about as much as in soft drinks. Even the "no added" sugar fruit juices, labelled as "natural" contain a lot of sugar.

Nor are "sugar free" diet drinks safe. Crichton, Alkerwi, and Elias (2015) showed that "diet" soft drinks were associated with MetS.

Conversely, Carrera-Lanestosa, Moguel-Ordóñez, and Segura-Campos (2017) showed that the natural sweetener, stevia (*Stevia rebaudiana Bertoni*) is able to treat MetS.

Peteliuk, Rybchuk, Bayliak, Storey, and Lushchak (2021) wrote that *"... biological activities of* S. rebaudiana *extract and its individual glycosides, including anti-hypertensive, anti-obesity, anti-diabetic, antioxidant, anti-cancer, anti-inflammatory, and antimicrobial effects and improvement of kidney function."*

To repeat, stevia can help treat MetS.

Kids watch advertisements on TV pushing all sorts of junk foods, from "health bars" to "healthy cereals" and, of course, fast food chains. Admittedly some are trying to clean up their acts by making salads and selling fruit. One chain is now brandishing the Heart Health tick. However, I am too sceptical and cynical to believe that a fast-food outlet deserves such an endorsement.

Harris, Pomeranz, Lobstein, and Brownell (2009) wrote that reducing food marketing to children is one way to reduce childhood obesity. However, *"significant social, legal, financial, and public perception barriers stand in the way. The scientific literature documents that food marketing to children is (a) massive; (b) expanding in number of venues (product placements, video games, the Internet, cell phones, etc.); (c) composed almost entirely of messages for nutrient-poor, calorie-dense foods; (d) having harmful effects; and (e) increasingly global and hence difficult to regulate by individual countries."*

Even the "sports drinks" are high in sugar *"for the energy"*!

What about the high sugar, chocolate covered bar that helps you "*work, rest and play!?"* It is interesting to note that the actors in these advertisements are all thin and healthy looking, giving the impression that these products are healthy: you hardly ever see obese actors promoting "healthy" obesogenic foods.

Children see these advertisements and believe the hype, i.e. that these products are healthy. So, they nag

Mum and Dad, and these foods are bought. Sometimes, even Mum and Dad think they are doing the healthy thing. Unfortunately, no. They are being duped.

Any altered food is bad; anything in a packet, tin or otherwise is not the best. Fresh food, cooked from scratch, is the best.

There was an advertisement a few years ago on TV which stated that "nine out of 10 nutritionists recommend a certain brand of cereal for breakfast." I must be that one out of ten, because I do not recommend cereal. It is probably the worst way to start the day. People are misled to believe that grains are good for them.

The human species has been on this earth for a very long time and grains were never a part of the diet until relatively recently.

Our species evolved (adapted) to a hunter-gatherer diet which is higher in animal protein and fats and lower in carbohydrates. We now eat a diet high in grains which our bodies have not adapted to. What do the orthodox dieticians and nutritionists tell us? Eat lots of grains.

What does the food pyramid show? Cereals and grains form the largest part of the recommended diet, but grains have never been a part of the human diet till recently.

Are grains healthy? There is a difference of opinion, and it seems to be a matter of degree. At one end of the spectrum is the highly refined white flour, which is made into white bread, white pasta, pastries, biscuits, cakes, etc. This is the terrible end of the spectrum. Most people will agree that these foods should be avoided.

Approximately in the middle of the spectrum are the whole grains. Studies show that they are healthy: but is this because they are compared to refined white products? So, we should say they are possibly healthier.

If you only eat refined white products and choose to change to whole grain, then there could be an improvement in your health. However, if you cut them out completely or minimize them, then the improvements may be even better.

The extreme other end of the spectrum is to eliminate grain completely from the diet. Grains, no matter how whole grained and unrefined, still are starchy and they contain gluten, a protein of wheat (and oats, barley, and rye) that can be toxic to humans.

Gluten is one factor that is generally not taken into consideration.

There are some who are *allergic* to gluten: this is

called coeliac disease. There is also a group who are not allergic but *intolerant* to gluten. It is remarkable how many people with digestive disorders, indigestion, bloating, constipation or diarrhoea, and excess flatulence, greatly improve after stopping all gluten containing food. In these people, gluten can possibly affect weight.

Freire et al. (2016) showed that in a mouse model, gluten intake increases weight and adiposity.

Soares et al. (2013) wrote *"Our data support the beneficial effects of gluten-free diets in reducing adiposity gain, inflammation and insulin resistance."* Again, this was in a mouse model.

What about humans?

The evidence is not as clear cut as in the animal models.

Brouns and Shewry (2022) discuss that in observational studies, gluten was not consistently related to body weight. The authors posit that if gluten is related to body weight, then countries with high gluten intake would have a higher incidence of overweight than countries with low gluten intake. This is not the case.

We can possibly conclude that in humans, gluten *per se* is probably not related to weight gain or loss.

However, it is obvious that by avoiding gluten containing products such as bread, cakes, biscuits, pastries, noodles, pasta, etc., you are also avoiding the sugar and the ultra-refined carbohydrates. Eating less of these foods can help with weight reduction.

On the other hand, gluten-free products tend to have more sugar (to make it taste better), but also less fibre, and more salt, and people tend to eat more which can lead to weight gain.

Another factor not considered are *phytates*. Phytates are substances found in grains and soy products that can bind minerals, such as Ca, Mg, iron (Fe), and zinc (Zn) and make them unavailable for absorption. Mineral deficiencies can occur in people who consume a high grain or soy diet. Phytates can be reduced by processes such as fermentation, soaking and sprouting (Gupta, Gangoliya, & Singh, 2015).

Sugar

Sugar is another issue that needs to be explored. If we look at our ancestral diet, there was very little, if any, sugar in the diet. Now it is a very large portion of the diet. Powell, Smith-Taillie, and Popkin (2016) wrote *"In 2011-2012, children and adults consumed 326 kcal/day and 308 kcal/day, respectively, of added sugars, or 14% and 17%, respectively, of total their energy."*

Unfortunately, humans can develop a "sweet tooth". This comes on very early in life: a baby introduced to sweetness early in life will develop this sweet tooth and then demand it, crave it - even become addicted to it.

Food manufacturers know this, so sugar is added. With the politically correct "low fat" foods, sugar is added to make them palatable.

Sugar is a cause of obesity: most people do not seem to realize this. They still think that it is the fat that makes you fat. People have been cutting out the fat and they are still getting fatter. Studies referenced throughout this book have shown this but, of course, the sugar industry denies the obvious.

Funny that.

A joint report released by the World Health Organization (WHO) and the Food and Agricultural Organization (FAO) in 2003 encouraged people to eat more fruit and vegetables and to limit the sugar to no more than 10% of the energy in the diet. (Personally, I think even that is too high!)

This was strongly contested when the US

ambassador to the FAO released a statement which basically said that the report was wrong. However, WH0 officials stood by their report. *"The report contains the best currently available scientific evidence on the relationship of diet, nutrition and physical activity to chronic disease."*

The US Sugar Association and other food industry groups reacted strongly to this limitation. They said that the report misleads the public to believe that there is a health risk (!) in consuming more than 10% of an individual's daily energy from added sugars!

There was great pressure on the WHO to prevent the release of the report, including a threat from the USA to withdraw the $406 million contribution to the WHO.

This is politics; this is economics and dollars, not health.

Of course, it is in the interests of the sugar manufacturers and the food industry groups to deny the WHO report findings. They make their profit by selling sugar.

In 2016, Kearns, Schmidt, and Glantz wrote "... *in 1965, a literature review was published in the New England Journal of Medicine, which singled out fat and cholesterol as the dietary causes of CHD and downplayed evidence that sucrose consumption was also a risk factor.", "Together with other recent analyses of sugar industry documents, our findings suggest the industry sponsored a research program in the 1960s and 1970s that successfully cast doubt about the hazards of sucrose while promoting fat as the dietary culprit in CHD."* (Emphasis the author)

The sugar industry has a lot to answer for.

Sugar is not healthy.

Ludwig, Peterson, and Gortmaker (2001) showed a direct correlation between obesity in children and the number of sugary drinks they consume.

Who do you believe?

The food and sugar industry that want to sell and make profit from the sale of sugar, or the scientists and nutritionists?

Marcus et al. (2009) reported on the Stockholm obesity prevention programme (STOPP). Schools were enlisted in Stockholm and divided into two groups. In one group, nutritious lunches (even though they consisted of low-fat dairy and whole grains) were encouraged and there was a ban on sweets, buns, and sweetened drinks. The other group did not introduce any specific rule.

The first group had a six percent drop in overweight children. In the schools where there were no such rules, the number of overweight children rose by three percent.

Just by changing lunches and banning sugary foods, the number of overweight children declined.

Then there are those nutritionists on TV who advertise foods. Investigate who pays them. If they are being paid, or sponsored by the manufacturer of the food, do not believe them.

In all these ways we are being mis-informed. We are being led to believe that these foods are "healthy" but on the contrary, they are doing us much harm. These high carbohydrate foods are a large part of the health and obesity problem. As I have already explained, the high carbohydrate/sugar foods stimulate insulin which leads to more fat storage.

Exercise

The food and sugar industry maintain that the obesity problem is not related to sugar but to a lack of exercise. Exercise has been shown to improve IR, the basic underlying metabolic defect in MetS.

An interesting question to pose is: Is it the diet? Or is it the lack of exercise? Which is more important?

We can argue back and forth but in reality, it is a combination of both.

I was watching the programme *"Extreme Makeover"* one night, (normally I don't watch that sort of thing!) and the physical training guru said something quite interesting. He said the weight loss was 80% diet and 20% exercise.

Our ancestors were very active, they had to be. Food could not be delivered to them like a dial a pizza: they had to run and hunt and carry their kill back to their caves. Hard physical activity. This is part of our physiology. But what is happening? We are very inactive. We sit in our car to go to work, we sit behind a computer all day, we drive back home, we sit and eat, we sit in front of the TV, then go to bed. Our modern technology is producing all sorts of "labour saving devices" which again reduce the activity we once engaged in.

There is less we have to do that requires physical energy.

Children do not play outside as much anymore; they sit indoors and play video games. There are many reasons for this. Some are related to poor urban planning, such as lack of playgrounds and lack of "green spaces". With increasing populations, the green spaces are being encroached upon by housing. Also with the increasing population, there is a great increase in traffic. Then there is the safety issue. Let's face it, there are a lot of crazy deviants lurking about. There is the fear of paedophiles. Murder, robbery, rape, kidnapping; many of these are unfortunately everyday events. With a society like that out there, no wonder parents are afraid to allow their children to go out, unsupervised.

Unsupervised is a keyword.

The parents are, of course, too busy to supervise, they must go to work. Today, the only way to survive is for both parents to work.

When I was a child in the 1960s, I walked or rode my bike to school, during recess breaks we played and ran about, and on weekends we wandered about all day and went back home for dinner: it was a much safer, perhaps even innocent, environment. But now, parents do not allow children to walk to school. They cannot roam about and play and explore, like I did in the 60s.

The world has changed completely.

Children sit at home in front of the TV, a truly "electronic babysitter." Children eat more while sitting in front of the TV than when outside playing.

Writing about the optimal diet is one thing. Doing it is another. Being able to afford it is an added complication.

Poverty is an issue becoming increasingly prevalent today: the gap between the "haves" and "have nots" is getting greater.

There are big contrasts.

In the third world where poverty is rife, there is just not enough food. Starvation is unfortunately too common.

In more developed nations, poverty is also an issue; the difference is that there is food available. There is no starvation but there is malnutrition. Unfortunately, the cheap foods are the unhealthier foods (Drewnowski & Specter 2004; Drewnowski & Darmon, 2005).

There are more and more families on a very tight budget. Housing, either rent or mortgage, is consuming a large percentage of income. This leads to financial stress. Less and less of the family income remains to purchase food, and unfortunately, the cheap foods are perhaps the unhealthiest: high in refined carbohydrates and sugars.

Other than the two more obvious factors, diet and (lack of) exercise, there are some influences generally not considered in the development of obesity. They are stress and lack of sleep, something we are all subject to in this modern world of ours. These could be the missing link in many with obesity. Many obese/overweight people diet, sweat, and exercise, yet still they do not lose weight. These two factors need to be considered when treating obesity. In fact, these two factors need to be considered when treating any facet of MetS.

Stress

As mentioned above, stress is a concern. We all know that stress is very common in this western, highly technological society we live in.

Stress is related to obesity.

On one level, some stressed people eat less (they are too stressed to eat!), however, for many, stress causes snacking, especially with "comfort foods" which tend to be high in sugars. Stress can make you feel hungry and therefore people tend to eat more. This, in itself, can lead to obesity.

Stress can cause obesity in other ways.

Yamaguchi et al. (2017) demonstrated that stress, particularly work stress, is a factor in the development of MetS and as we now know, obesity is one of the symptoms of MetS.

Serrano Ríos (2005) suggested that MetS is a modern variant of the stress-related disorder.

Stress causes the release of cortisol, the stress hormone, which is known to encourage fat accumulation. The connection may not be that simple: studies have shown conflicting results. Perhaps cortisol is not the only player: it is a very complex situation.

Stress also has a direct influence on metabolism, which in turn influences weight and fat accumulation. When stressed, the body releases a molecule, neuropeptide Y (NPY), which has an impact on the fat cells, encouraging and boosting them to grow in size and number (Kuo et al., 2007).

Sleep

As we have seen, the modern population sleeps much less than our ancestors did. We evolved with a day/night circadian rhythm and a disruption to this will cause disease.

Reduced sleep is linked to the development of MetS and obesity (Vorona et al., 2005; Gohil & Hannon, 2018).

Studies of shift workers, compared to day workers, show an increased incidence of obesity, high triglycerides, and low HDL levels (Karlsson, Knutsson, & Lindahl, 2001).

In women, there may be an association between shift work and breast cancer (Gehlert & Clanton, 2020). This indicates a relationship between the sleep disruption from shift work, melatonin and MetS.

Obesity is just a symptom, a symptom of a distorted metabolic problem. Increasing exercise is an important part of the equation but just as important, perhaps even more so, is a change in diet. A healthy diet must include more vegetables, salads, fruits, nuts, meats, and eggs and fewer sugars and other refined carbohydrates. Conventional wisdom says it is the fats but, in reality, it is more the sugars.

And so, it is clear that other factors such as stress and lack of sleep must be considered when treating obesity.

DIABETES

"The doctor of the future will give no medicine but will interest his patients in the care of the human frame, in diet and in the cause and prevention of disease."
Thomas Edison (1847 – 1931)

Diabetes is another manifestation of MetS.

Diabetes is not just a disease of blood sugar levels (BSL). Diabetes is a result of an abnormal underlying metabolism. Here again, is it enough to just deal with the superficial manifestations? To just "reduce the numbers"? Or is it best to deal with the underlying problem that caused the sugar level to go up in the first place? Ideally, treatment should include some of both.

Types of diabetes

There are two main types of diabetes: type 1 (T1D) and type 2 (T2D), though other forms can be considered.

T1D is often called juvenile onset diabetes mellitus (JODM), or insulin dependent diabetes mellitus (IDDM). This type of diabetes occurs when the pancreatic cells that produce insulin are destroyed by an autoimmune process.

T2D is often referred to as mature onset diabetes mellitus (MODM), or non-insulin dependent diabetes mellitus (NIDDM).

I will mostly discuss T2D as it is more common and is related to MetS. The explosion of diabetes that is seen in western society is largely the T2D variety.

Type 3 diabetes is related to Alzheimer's disease (AD) and is often referred to as "diabetes of the brain".

"Studies suggesting AD as a metabolic disease caused by insulin resistance in the brain also offer strong support for the hypothesis that AD is a type 3 diabetes" (Michailidis et al., 2022).

Alzheimer's disease will be discussed later.

Type 3c diabetes is a term used where the pancreas is damaged and therefore cannot produce insulin. This includes conditions such as acute or chronic pancreatitis, pancreatic cancer, cystic fibrosis, haemochromatosis, and where the pancreas has been surgically removed (pancreatectomy).

Gestational diabetes mellitus (GDM) is another type of diabetes. This is the diabetes of pregnancy. In many cases, women who develop GDM are obese and may eventually develop T2D, and as such, it is related to IR and MetS.

T2D is a big issue; increasing numbers of people are developing this condition and no longer can it be called "mature onset" because the age at which this condition develops is getting younger and younger. We now have pre-pubertal children developing a disease which, up until recently, developed only in the elderly. Frightening, isn't it?

Before we go any further, giving a definition of diabetes is probably a good idea. Shaw and Chisholm (2003) defined T2D as *"...a complex metabolic disorder characterised by hyperglycaemia and associated with a relative deficiency of insulin secretion, along with a reduced response of target tissues to insulin (insulin resistance)."*

I have only one criticism about this definition. I disagree with *"a relative deficiency of insulin secretion"* because in T2D, the pancreas is usually very good at high secretion of insulin, the levels of insulin can be high, and the problem is that the tissues do not respond. That is the IR. Though eventually the pancreas may fail.

So, why is there so much diabetes these days?

I think if you have read the book thus far, you probably can answer the question. Yes: it is mostly due to a disordered metabolism caused by diet and lifestyle not suited to the human species.

Again, we go back to our ancestral diet. Generally higher in protein, fat, vegetables, salads, fruits, nuts, berries and very low in sugar, and very low in refined carbohydrates, and grains.

But what is our western diet now? High in sugars, refined carbohydrates and low in fats and proteins.

This is just a repetition of what I have already said.

T2D should be considered in context. It is not an isolated condition: it is very closely related to obesity, heart disease, hypertension, and cholesterol. Should the symptoms (conditions) be treated individually, or should the underlying metabolic problem be addressed? Or both?

We should treat the superficial conditions, i.e. "reduce the numbers" but we must also address the underlying metabolic issue.

We know the condition is becoming increasingly common.

The incidence of T2D increased almost 3-fold (from 400,000 to 1.2 million between 2000 and 2021. So that in Australia in 2001, almost 4.6% of the population was living with T2D. It was 1.3 times more likely to occur in males than females.

(https://www.aihw.gov.au › reports › diabetes › diabetes-australian-facts › contents › how-common-is-diabetes/type-2-diabetes - Accessed 13 August 2023)

Fox et al. (2006) reported on a doubling of incidence of T2D between the 1970s to the 1990s.

The fact that the incidence of diabetes has grown faster than the population growth shows that something in the modern lifestyle is causing it. By dealing with this lifestyle issue, the problem should therefore be prevented.

What is so bad about the western diet?

If you have read the book to this point, you will know it is the unhealthy, high, refined carbohydrate diet. Most concerning is that the powers that be are actually encouraging this unhealthy diet.

"Increasing intakes of refined carbohydrate (corn syrup) concomitant with decreasing intakes of fibre paralleled the upward trend in the prevalence of type 2 diabetes observed in the United States during the 20th Century" (Gross, Li, Ford, & Liu, 2004).

One of the worst factors is sugar. Sugar is put into nearly all manufactured foods. Politically correct, "low fat" foods are being made and heavily promoted. People are encouraged to be afraid of fat; they are encouraged to think that low fat is better, so they buy "low fat" products. How correct is this? Is it really healthier?

The problem is that when fat is removed, the taste goes. So, what is put in its place to give it taste? Answer … sugar. This cannot possibly be healthier.

Does sugar cause diabetes?

The information can be confusing, even complicated.

If you search the internet, you will find many sites that state very clearly that sugar does not "directly" cause diabetes. Although they do say sugar is "associated" with T2D. I think it is important you have a close look at who supports these sites: Is it the sugar industry, some "foundation" or some food manufacturer? These bodies obviously have a vested interest. Their profit comes from selling sugar, so I do not think they will tell you not to buy any! There is a conflict of interest.

There are some other sites that "sit on the fence" … are a bit more neutral. They say that sugar does not cause T2D (they are probably being 'politically correct") but they also say that it may be a "contributing factor"; such as sugar can cause obesity that could lead to T2D.

Excess sugar and refined carbohydrates stimulate insulin excessively and eventually lead to IR which can lead to T2D.

In the past, the sugar industry liked to quote one particular study; Black et al. (2006). The conclusion was that *"In this study, a high-sucrose intake as part of an eucaloric, weight-maintaining diet had no detrimental effect on insulin sensitivity, glycemic profiles, or measures of vascular compliance in healthy nondiabetic subjects."*

A close look at this study showed that the study was done on thirteen healthy volunteers for six weeks. Hardly a huge study. The problem is not what sugar does in a six-week period but what it does over years.

So, does eating lots of sugar and refined carbohydrates lead to diabetes?

There are many studies that show an association

between sugar consumption and T2D (Wang, Yu, Fang, & Hu, 2015; Imamura et al., 2015).

Weeratunga, Jayasinghe, Perera, Jayasena, and Jayasinghe (2014) showed a strong positive correlation between prevalence of T2D and per capita sugar consumption.

Sugar is known to increase body weight and increase fat storage which can lead to T2D.

Vasselli, Scarpace, Harris, and Banks (2013) described animal studies which show that large sugar intake can disrupt leptin signalling, which can lead to overeating and weight gain.

Weight gain/obesity is related to MetS.

Before we go any further, it is important to introduce the concept of the glycaemic index.

The glycaemic index (GI) is a ranking system for carbohydrates based on their effect on blood sugar levels in the first two hours. It compares carbohydrates gram for gram in individual foods, providing a numerical, evidence-based index of postprandial (post-meal) glycaemia (Ciok & Dolna, 2006).

Carbohydrates that break down slowly, releasing glucose gradually into the bloodstream, have a low GI.

A lower GI suggests slower rates of digestion and absorption of the sugars. A lower glycaemic response is often thought to equate to a lower insulin demand, better long-term blood sugar control and a reduction in blood lipids.

It is important not to consider carbohydrates in terms of simple or complex but rather in terms of GI. In general, the lower the GI, the better. Some examples are, gram dal 7, peanuts 21, soya beans 25, cherries 32, red lentils 36, chickpeas 47, apple 54, pinto beans 55, orange 63, instant boiled rice 65, fruit loaf 67, chocolate 70, kiwifruit 75, sweet corn 78, boiled potato 80, wheat bread 99, carrots 101, pumpkin 107, jellybeans 114, baked potato 121.

As with everything else, there are exceptions. Some low GI foods can cause other problems. For example, fructose has a GI of only 32. It does not convert to glucose and raise blood sugar levels; rather it converts to triglycerides in the liver. This is probably the reason why people who eat a lot of fruit have high serum triglycerides.

Another concept to consider is the glycaemic load (GL). This looks at the actual content of carbohydrates based on the carbohydrate content and portion size (Venn & Green, 2007). This fine-tunes the concept of the GI. For example, some foods may have a relatively high

GI, yet the amount of carbohydrate may be low. The GL can be calculated as the quantity of carbohydrate in grams multiplied by the GI and divided by 100.

If we look at the western diet, we can see that, generally, it is a relatively high GI and a high GL diet. That is, excess refined carbohydrates, and high in sugar that raises the blood sugar levels easily and quickly. This elicits a robust insulin response and, in the long term, has a role in the development of the IR, which we have discussed previously.

So, in effect, it is not specifically that a high GI diet causes diabetes; it causes IR, and diabetes is a symptom of the hyperinsulinaemia/IR syndrome, which we know as MetS.

DiNicolantonio and O'Keefe (2022) showed that added dietary sugars drive IR, hyperinsulinaemia, hypertension, T2D, heart disease and obesity, i.e. MetS.

The population is eating increasingly larger amounts of sugar. In the majority of cases this is because the sugar is added to the manufactured food products. Next time you go to the supermarket, have a look at any product and examine the food composition table on the packet. It will be a challenge to find a product that contains no sugar.

Food manufacturers have also been very naughty.

Russell, Baker, Grimes, Lindberg, and Lawrence (2023) looked at the sugar content of food. They showed that over the years, food manufacturers had initially been increasing the amount of added sugar, but with government push to reduce sugar content of food, they reduced the sugar and substituted with "non-nutritive sweeteners" (NNS), defined as *"substances with little to no energy which impart sweetness."* However, observational studies have reported associations between NNS consumption and weight gain, changes to the gut microbiome and T2D.

These NNS include:

- aspartame
- cyclamate
- erythritol
- mannitol
- sorbitol
- xylitol.

This list also includes stevia, which has been discussed earlier.

However, in the less developed countries, the food manufacturers have continued to increase the amount of sugar.

Most of the population is eating too much sugar.

One survey, published in *Vaccination Roulette* (1989) by the Australian Vaccination Network, looked at the most popular items that people are buying from the supermarkets in Australia.

These are, in order:

1. Coca-Cola 375mls,
2. Coca-Cola 1 litre,
3. Coca-Cola 2 litres,
4. Diet coke 375mls,
5. Cherry ripe,
6. Nestle's condensed milk,
7. Tally Ho cigarette papers,
8. Mars bars,
9. Kit Kat,
10. Crunchie bar,
11. Eta 5-star margarine,
12. Heinz baked beans,
13. Golden circle tinned beetroot,
14. Bushell's tea,
15. Diet coke 1 litre,
16. Cadbury milk chocolate,
17. Pepsi cola 375mls,
18. Coca-Cola 1.5 litres,
19. Kellogg's corn flakes,
20. Maggie 2-minute noodles (chicken

flavour),
21. Generic brand lemon drink,
22. Panadol tablets (24 pack),
23. Meadow Lea margarine.

A similar survey was done in 2023 (from the USA; and Australia is probably not much different).

1. Soda (Coke, Sprite) & soft drinks
2. Milk
3. Chips (Chitos, Doritos & Lay's)
4. Eggs
5. Bread
6. Breakfast cereals & instant oatmeal
7. Candy bars (Kit Kat, Snickers & Milky way etc.)
8. Block cheese & Deli cheese
9. Beer
10. Bottled water
11. Cigarettes & e-cigarettes. Also, tobacco and lighters.
12. Chocolate bars
13. Snack cakes, e.g., the likes of Debbie, Reese's, Hostess.
14. Cookies and crackers. Primarily similar ones to Oreo.
15. Pepperoni, jerky, bacon, ham & other packaged meats

16. Wine
17. Cupcakes and muffins
18. Breakfast bars & granola bars
19. Fresh fruits (esp. bananas, apples & lemons) The other most popular and profitable products to sell will also be blueberries. Bananas are one of the most purchased products in the U.S. and the most purchased fruit in the U.S. Another top selling fruit is oranges.
20. Fresh vegetables (esp. potatoes, tomatoes & cucumber)

(https://businessnes.com/list-of-top-selling-grocery-items-and-tips/ - Accessed 14 August 2023)

Consider that list. Not much has changed, although fruit and vegetables are included in the more recent list.

So, I ask again. Does eating excess sugar, which is itself a high calorie diet, high GI diet, cause diabetes?

Yes!

Salmerón et al. (1997) studied 65,173 healthy women, aged 40 to 65 who were followed over a six-year period. Out of these, 915 developed T2D. The study concluded that dietary GI was positively associated with risk of diabetes, after adjustment for age, body mass index, smoking, physical activity, family history of diabetes, alcohol and cereal fibre intake, and total energy intake.

In a parallel study, Salmerón et al. (1997) studied 42,759 men, free of diabetes and heart disease, between the ages of 45 and 75 years. They were followed for six years. As with the women, a high GI diet was positively associated with the development of T2D.

These findings have been confirmed by newer studies (Oba et al., 2013; Willett, Manson, & Liu, 2002).

In the western world, perhaps one of the highest intakes of sugar comes from the consumption of sugar-laden soft drinks. To this we could add fruit juices, which are advertised as "healthy" but are high in sugar. It is quite easy to drink a litre of orange juice, but could you eat 20-30 oranges? Possibly not but you could drink the sugar from that number of oranges very easily. People rationalize that because fruit and fruit juice are "healthy" they can eat and drink unlimited quantities, get their sweet fix and still be "healthy".

Sugar containing drinks contribute to obesity and to T2D. The data comes from the Harvard Nurses' Health II Study. Schulze et al. (2004) found that higher consumption of sugar-sweetened beverages was associated with an increased magnitude of weight gain and a development of T2D.

Soft drinks (or as the Americans call it “soda” or “pop”) are a huge source of sugar. The USA is the second highest consumer of soft drink per year; 154 litres/capita (the highest is Argentina at 155 litres/capita).

(https://worldpopulationreview.com › country-rankings › soda-consumption-by-country - Accessed 2 December 2023)

Australia was not in the top 10 countries.

In 1900, the average annual consumption was about twelve bottles per person. In the late 1950s it had increased to 150 bottles per person.

This trend continued to increase.

Americans consumed 15.25 billion gallons of soft drink in 1999. This makes soft drinks America’s favourite refreshment exceeding tea, coffee and juice combined. This averages out to 56 gallons per person per year, which accounts for nearly a quarter of daily calorie intake.

To put the above into perspective, White (2018) showed that the amount of sugar in just one standard 16-oz soda (“pop”, soft drink) is 64 grams or 16 teaspoons.

In 2004, Americans spent $37 billion on

carbonated beverages alone.

Another excuse that is commonly bandied about is that sugar does not cause diabetes, but obesity causes diabetes (but then, sugar can cause obesity). As we have already discussed, sugar, and other refined carbohydrates cause obesity. To tie this all together, we should not look at the superficial manifestations, i.e. obesity or diabetes, but the underlying metabolism. This refined high sugar, western diet, causes MetS which manifests as obesity and/or diabetes.

Another argument used; and I think this is done to get the spotlight off sugar is to blame fat.

Fat has been blamed for a long time. Everyone "knows" that fat is bad, fat puts on weight, fat causes heart disease, fat causes diabetes. As we have previously seen, the sugar industry paid scientists to move the focus off sugar and onto fat.

Unfortunately, people believe what they see on TV and/or hear on radio. The average person's knowledge of nutrition comes from advertisements in the media. The advertisements do not teach proper nutrition. Advertisements are there to sell products.

So, if you believe the advertisements and that includes the "dietician" or the "nutritionist" who promotes certain produce - be suspicious. This is not nutritional education. It is propaganda to sell that product.

Fat does not necessarily make you fat.

This is not what the average person knows. They think eating fat makes you fat.

This is partly because of the large number of "low fat" products.

When indoctrinated to believe fat is bad, then the population will buy the "low fat" products.

My counter argument is that despite eating "low fat" products, people continue to get fatter.

The human species has been eating fat for centuries. Obesity has only become a problem in the last 60 - 70 years or so.

One issue is probably the form of fat. There is the good and the bad, and possibly the ugly. Unfortunately, it is the bad and ugly fats that have given fat a bad name. The worst fats are *trans* fatty acids (TFAs).

Some TFAs do occur in nature, but the quantities are extremely small. The largest source of TFAs is processed foods, especially margarine, as well as commercial fried foods and bakery products which are made with shortening, margarine, or partially hydrogenated oil. Such products include crackers, cookies, doughnuts, pastries, muffins, croissants, snack foods and fried foods, such as French fries and breaded foods.

How much of the western diet is included in that list?

In a large proportion of cases, in the process of trying to avoid fat, people tend to increase their intake of TFAs.

Diabetes has also been blamed on fat. This again is possibly to take the spotlight off sugar and other refined carbohydrates.

Unfortunately, it is not specifically the fat that may cause diabetes, it is the TFAs. Salmerón et al. (2001) wrote that *"The data suggests that total fat and saturated and monounsaturated fatty intakes are not associated with risk of type 2 diabetes in women, but that trans fatty acids increase and poly unsaturated fatty acids reduce risk."*

So, all those people who eat out, who eat at fast food restaurants, are eating a large amount of TFAs.

Obesity is a risk factor for diabetes. That is true.

Even mainstream doctors agree with that.

Also generally accepted is that losing weight will improve diabetes. Again, true, and again, accepted by mainstream doctors. However, reducing dietary fat is not the way to go. Reducing fat will not necessarily reduce obesity. Reducing fat will probably exacerbate the situation.

The idea does sound logical, reduce the fat in your diet and you will lose weight. To some extent, if you are eating a diet with excess fats, then some reduction may help. The worst combination is eating excess fats with excess carbohydrates. However, generally, reducing fat more will not help and may be counterproductive. Fat is an essential part of human nutrition, even the saturated fats, which have been so demonised. Saturated fats have been a part of human nutrition for a very long time and obesity and diabetes have only been a major issue for about the last 60 - 70 years.

Also, statistics have shown that the dietary intake of fat has been decreasing, yet we are getting fatter and developing more diabetes. So, just from that it can be seen that fat is not a cause. By reducing fat, what happens? You still must eat. A low-fat diet tastes bland, so, to make it palatable, sugar is added. Also, fat is satisfying, and it curbs the appetite. By eating more fat, you become more satisfied and overall eat less.

By reducing the fat, just the opposite happens. You are less satisfied, and you tend to eat more. You eat your "low fat" product, and you eat the whole packet because they are: -

1. not satisfying and
2. are "low fat" therefore you think it is "healthy" (but it is high in sugar).

People rationalise that they are therefore healthy and wonder why things are getting worse.

The artificial sweeteners are no better. Besides the side effects and toxic action of these chemicals, they do not necessarily help to lose weight. When one of these artificial sweeteners is used, you may fool the tongue, but this does not fool the brain: the tendency is to eat more and therefore gain weight.

Diabetes can be controlled, prevented, and dare I say it, cured by increasing protein and fat and reducing sugars, starches, and carbohydrates, as well as by improving the lifestyle.

The study below highlights the situation where starches and sugar have been reduced and replaced by fat. The result was a loss of weight and an improvement in heart disease markers, such as cholesterol and triglycerides, thus negating the assumption that a high fat diet causes heart disease.

Hays, Gorman, and Shakir (2002) wrote *"Addition of saturated fat and removal of starch from a high mono-unsaturated fat and starch restricted diet improved glycaemia control and were associated with weight loss without detectable adverse effects on serum lipids."*

The typical US diet is high in glycaemic load: 18.6% comes from sugars, syrups, and honey and another 20.4% comes from refined cereal grains. In total, over 39% of the total dietary energy comes from foods that were virtually never found in the ancestral diet.

Exercise

We have become a very sedentary lot. We sit on our backsides most of the day. In contrast, our ancestors were very active; they had to be just to survive.

Joseph et al. (2019) showed that exercise is a very important aspect in the prevention and treatment of, not just diabetes, but MetS in general, which includes obesity.

The basic effect of exercise is to improve the function of the muscles. The muscles are like a sugar sponge: continued moderate exercise will increase muscle glucose uptake by 20 times the normal rate. Although it is not yet known how, it is known that exercise will help to improve the IR (Whillier, 2020).

Church (2011) noted that; *"The risk of developing both metabolic syndrome and type 2 diabetes mellitus (T2DM) is inversely associated with regular exercise training."*

Exercise will also help with weight loss, improves bone density, lowers blood pressure and it gets you out of the house into the sunshine where the vitamin D factor will be improved.

The cheapest and easiest form of exercise is walking.

"Walking is a man's best medicine."
Hippocrates (c460-c370 BCE)

Sleep

We have already seen that a lack of sleep can cause health problems. A lack of sleep can predispose to MetS. This of course includes diabetes.

Ayas et al. (2003) showed that *"Sleep restriction may be an independent factor for developing symptomatic diabetes."*

Yaggi, Araujo, and McKinlay (2006) concluded that *"Short and long sleep durations increase the risk of developing diabetes, independent of confounding factors. Sleep duration may represent a novel risk factor for diabetes."* They showed that too short (less than six hours a night) or too long (greater than eight hours a night) sleep are risk factors for developing diabetes.

The men in this study were grouped into five categories, according to length of sleep. 1) less than or equal to five hours, 2) six hours, 3) seven hours, 4) eight hours and 5) greater than eight hours. Those who slept less than five hours and six hours a night was twice as likely to develop diabetes, while those who slept more than eight hours were three times more likely to develop diabetes over the study follow-up period of 5-7 years.

So, again, to treat diabetes, as all the other symptoms of MetS, we must not only look at the diet but must consider other life-style factors as well, including sleep, stress, exercise, and sunshine.

CHOLESTEROL

"'Listen, Doc,' he went on, sounding worried. 'There's something I've been wanting to ask you for a long time. Where could I get my blood cholesterol measured?'

'Your what?!'..........'You're far more likely to fall down a hatch and break your neck.' "

From **Doctor at Sea**, by Richard Gordon.

For many years, cholesterol was a word that meant little to the average person, and then in a very short space of time, it has become a topic of conversation on everyone's lips.

We have been taught to fear cholesterol.

All we hear is "cholesterol is dangerous".

How correct is this?

Mainstream doctors are telling their patients to get

their cholesterol levels checked and to reduce the levels as low as possible to protect them from heart disease. They believe that high cholesterol leads to heart disease, heart attacks, strokes, and death. They advise their patients to lower their cholesterol levels: the lower the better.

However, there are doctors who do not think that cholesterol is as big an issue as is made out. They feel that the cholesterol issue is being overemphasized. Some even say that there is no connection between cholesterol and heart disease.

Ravnskov et al. (2018) wrote that there is no evidence that the "bad" cholesterol causes heart disease, and that statins (drugs that reduce cholesterol levels) treatment is of "doubtful benefit".

The diet heart hypothesis, also known as the cholesterol hypothesis, began when Nikolai Anichkov (also spelled Anitschkow) (1885 – 1964) in 1913 undertook an experiment where he fed cholesterol to rabbits, and they developed atherosclerosis. This may not be valid, as rabbits are vegetarian and feeding cholesterol to vegetarian rabbits is using an inappropriate animal model. The same experiment was carried out using other animals that were carnivores; the same results were not able to be reproduced. Later, in the 1950s, Ancel Keys (1904 – 2004) published his Seven

Country Study. This showed a correlation between fat/cholesterol intake and heart disease. It seems he “cherry picked” the countries, as he had data from many other countries, but selected only those countries where the correlation could be made. From this came the hypothesis that fat and cholesterol intake lead to atherosclerosis which leads to cardiovascular disease and death.

After Keys’ purported discovery, the mantra became “eat less fat and cholesterol” to prevent heart disease. Various health departments, heart societies and other medical societies jumped on the bandwagon and for the last 60 - 70 years it has been “eat less fat”.

The drug companies also became involved: through researching and making drugs to lower cholesterol. The early cholesterol lowering drugs did lower blood cholesterol levels but there was minimal change in heart deaths. Although, when statins were first introduced, they seemed to work.

However, in a review of 35 randomised trials of cholesterol lowering by DuBroff, Malhotra and de Lorgeril (2021), they found no benefit for statin use achieving the cholesterol targets. They questioned the validity of using LDL cholesterol as a surrogate target for the prevention of heart disease.

The researchers looked at trials that reduced cholesterol by over 50% and there was no effect on mortality, while other trials showed only a 11-15% drop but had significant improvement in mortality.

It seems that any benefit is not from lowering cholesterol itself.

> *"However, a few supportive studies cannot outweigh the large number of contradictory ones"*
> (Ravnskov, 2008).

Or are there other factors which need to be explored.

The standard protocol

To lower cholesterol, medical authorities recommend trying dietary means before using medication. Mainstream doctors first tell patients to change their diet. They are then told that if the levels don't go down, they will need to go on a stricter diet and then, ultimately, a drug.

My first concern is the diet that these patients are asked to follow. The recommended diet will probably make things worse.

Ask any mainstream doctor: *"What diet do you recommend to patients to lower the cholesterol levels?"* Their probable answer is to avoid all fat and cholesterol. Cut out eggs and reduce meat and trim off all the fat as well as eat more grains and cereals. Eat low fat. Eat the "low fat" products. Eat more vegetables.

After a three month follow up the levels are still high, so they say, with regret, that the diet did not work. A drug is then prescribed.

For a start, the dietary advice is wrong. Following a diet like that will not lower cholesterol. Research over a very long time has shown that there is little direct correlation between dietary cholesterol and serum cholesterol. Lowering the cholesterol in the diet will not lower serum cholesterol significantly.

Perhaps those mainstream doctors do not know any better. Even worse, perhaps they were given the wrong advice. After all, if the proper diet was followed, cholesterol levels can go down and patients will not have to go on a drug. However, diet does not provide profits for the drug companies. Is it possible this erroneous advice is given on purpose?

Perhaps I am a sceptic!

One question that is essential to ask: Where do mainstream doctors get their dietary information from? Answer: the drug companies. What literature do these doctors give their patients? More than likely, they give patients information produced by a drug company, or perhaps some “independent” foundation. I used inverted commas because if you look hard enough, there will be some drug company connection to that “independent” foundation.

How convenient! Recommend a diet that does not work so that they can be put on a drug.

We should get back to basics.

Consider the human diet over the last couple of hundred thousand years. Humans are not vegetarians: they are omnivores. They will eat anything. Meat, fat and therefore cholesterol were a large part of the hunter-gatherer diet. Some researchers estimate that up to 65% of the paleolithic diet was from animal sources and as we all know, cholesterol occurs only in food from animal sources. This, for a start, does not make sense. Our ancestral diet is high in fat, cholesterol, and protein. Why should cholesterol in our diet suddenly become a problem? Humans must have developed/evolved some form of mechanism to deal with cholesterol. The cholesterol issue did not become prominent until only about 60 years ago and, if what we are told is true, i.e. cholesterol is a killer, then humanity should have become extinct centuries ago.

Perhaps it is some other component of the diet?

Or are there other factors involved?

The current dogma states that cholesterol in our diet gets into our blood which then clogs up our arteries and then we have heart attacks and die. This is what the average doctor knows because this is what they have been told.

How true is this?

Unfortunately, this is largely wrong.

Cholesterol does not necessarily cause heart disease.

Cholesterol is not necessarily the problem.

The problem is not that cholesterol levels are high, but rather, the issue is what causes cholesterol levels to rise.

Cholesterol is a marker.

I have already mentioned the car analogy. Do you fiddle with the temperature gauge to show a lower temperature? Or do you stop and look at the engine to determine why the temperature went up?

Lowering cholesterol levels is like fiddling with the temperature gauge. It does nothing to alter the underlying metabolism that causes the cholesterol to go up. The underlying metabolism is probably also the cause of heart disease.

We are continually being told to reduce cholesterol in our diet. An important question to ask is: *"Does dietary cholesterol cause serum cholesterol level to go up?"*

The answer is *"Only minimally"*.

Dietary cholesterol only marginally raises blood cholesterol levels, and this does not necessarily cause heart disease. There are many papers in many journals to show this, e.g., Soliman (2018), Ravnskov et al. (2018). Many mainstream doctors do not necessarily read journals; they rely mainly on drug company literature.

We are told to avoid fat and cholesterol and eggs because they contain cholesterol. But is this correct?

It is correct that the foods do contain cholesterol but does dietary cholesterol end up in the bloodstream?

Even the Reader's Digest knows better!

The cover from the Australian Reader's Digest, Sept 2004, says *"Eggs have little effect on serum cholesterol"* and *"No link between egg consumption and CVD"* (CVD = cardiovascular disease). Who can ignore the Reader's Digest?

Yet we have been told for years that we shouldn't eat eggs because they contain cholesterol, and they will raise your serum cholesterol and cause heart disease. Doctors have been limiting their patients to one egg a week.

The Tecumseh Study, in 1976, Nichols, Ravenscroft, Lamphiear, and Ostrander (1976) attempted to correlate blood cholesterol levels with the amounts of cholesterol and fat eaten. No positive correlation was found. *"Cholesterol and triglyceride levels were unrelated to quality, quantity, or proportions of fat, carbohydrate, or protein consumed in the 24-hr recall period."*

A similar relationship was found in the famous Framingham Study.

William Castelli, the director of the Framingham

Study wrote in 1992: *"In Framingham, Mass, the more saturated fat one ate, the more cholesterol one ate, the more calories one ate, the lower the person's serum cholesterol......we found that the people who ate the most cholesterol, ate the most saturated fat, ate the most calories, weighed the least and were the most physically active"*.

The research shows an inverse relationship between dietary cholesterol and serum cholesterol.

I have tried this in clinical practice. I have put people on a higher protein, fat, cholesterol and lower carbohydrate diet and surprise, surprise, their serum cholesterol went down.

I should point out a few things here.

- A higher fat/cholesterol/protein diet is our ancestral diet. This is the diet our ancestors lived on.
- A higher protein/fat diet means, usually, a lower carbohydrate diet.

An interesting question is: "Is it the higher cholesterol or is it the lower carbohydrates?" Or perhaps a bit of both?

The body makes most of the cholesterol, only about 20% comes from diet. So here we can say that dietary cholesterol only has a minimal impact. The rate limiting step in cholesterol synthesis is mediated by the enzyme *3-hydroxy-3-methylglutaryl CoA reductase* (HMG CoA reductase).

Insulin stimulates HMGCoA reductase activity. Other hormones such as oestrogen and thyroid hormone also influence this enzyme's expression, while glucocorticoids reduce. Thyroid hormone can increase HMGCoA reductase activity, and paradoxically, a thyroid hormone deficiency can also increase activity, hence the elevated levels of cholesterol in hypothyroidism (Ness & Chambers, 2000).

The simplicity of the system is that if the diet is high in carbohydrates, and therefore low or nil in cholesterol, the high insulin levels stimulate the production of cholesterol, because there is none in the diet. Conversely, when there is plenty of protein and fat, glucagon, the opposite of insulin, is stimulated, and this switches off the HMGCoA reductase because there is assumedly plenty of cholesterol in the diet.

Therefore, a high sugar/high carbohydrate diet increases insulin levels, which then increases cholesterol production.

The expression of this enzyme is inhibited by cholesterol (and by statin drugs), meaning that as cholesterol levels go up from absorption, the endogenous synthesis is reduced (Soliman, 2018).

Gylling et al. (2010) demonstrated the effect of IR on this mechanism. Cholesterol synthesis is upregulated, and absorption is downregulated in IR, which includes obesity, T2D, i.e. MetS.

According to Eddy, Schlessinger, Kahn, Peskin, and Schiebinger (2009), IR is the most important single cause of coronary artery disease (CAD).

Another interesting fact about cholesterol is that, although the body can make it, it cannot break it down. Cholesterol can only be removed from the body intact in the bile. This emphasises the need for good liver function, good bile production, good bowel actions and a high fibre diet to prevent re-absorption of the cholesterol.

The mean dietary cholesterol intake was 293 mg/day (348 mg/day for men and 242 mg/day for women) in the 2013-2014 National Health and Nutrition Examination Surveys (NHANES) (Xu, McClure, & Appel, 2018). On average, only about half of the cholesterol in the gut is absorbed and the rest is eliminated in the faeces (Cohn, Kamili, Wat, Chung, & Tandy, 2010).

Le Roy et al. (2019) demonstrated that the gut microbiota is involved in the absorption of cholesterol. Here is another reason to keep your gut microbiota happy.

Cholesterol is an essential nutrient: it is the starting point for many steroid hormones, including the sex hormones, cortisol, and vitamin D.

The waxy properties of cholesterol are needed to keep cell membranes firm and watertight.

A large proportion of the brain is composed of cholesterol. The insulating structure around the nerves, called the myelin sheath, is largely cholesterol. Animal studies showed that blocking cholesterol metabolism interferes with myelin formation (Saher et al., 2005).

Cholesterol is important.

Cholesterol is an essential nutrient.

When a patient responds to advice to eat less cholesterol, what happens? The body senses that there is less cholesterol coming in, so it starts to make more.

Conversely, by increasing the dietary cholesterol,

the body senses that there is adequate cholesterol, so the cholesterol making machinery in the liver is switched down.

This makes sense.

People are very surprised when I advise them to eat more cholesterol, especially when their “problem” is high cholesterol. Initially they are sceptical, but after a few months and a repeat test, which invariably shows a decreased cholesterol level, they are convinced. They are surprised that they are eating more cholesterol, yet their serum cholesterol is lower.

When people eat a higher protein/fat/cholesterol diet, they invariably eat fewer sugars, grains, and refined carbohydrates. Of course, grains, sugars, and refined carbohydrates were never a part of the ancestral diet.

Sugars have been shown to reduce the “good cholesterol” and increase the “bad cholesterol”. DiNicolantonio, Lucan, and O'Keefe (2016) wrote *“When saturated fats are replaced with refined carbohydrates, and specifically with added sugars (like sucrose or high fructose corn syrup), the end result is not favorable for heart health. Such replacement leads to changes in LDL, high-density lipoprotein (HDL), and triglycerides that may increase the risk of CHD.”*

The current theory: A high cholesterol, high fat

diet causes the serum cholesterol to go up which causes heart disease. Sounds simple, doesn't it?

In reality it is much more complicated.

So far, we have seen that dietary cholesterol and fat have little connection with serum cholesterol, therefore reducing dietary cholesterol will not necessarily lower serum cholesterol.

Eating cholesterol does not raise serum cholesterol.

Does cholesterol cause heart disease?

The mainstream must think so, because they spend a great deal of time and effort trying to reduce serum cholesterol.

They assume that since the arteries are clogged up with cholesterol, therefore cholesterol is the cause. This may sound logical but is it true?

High cholesterol may be a risk factor, but risk factors are not necessarily the cause.

Risk factors are not a disease.

If high serum cholesterol causes heart diseases, then it must follow that those who have higher cholesterol levels have more atherosclerotic arteries than those with lower cholesterol levels. This has never been shown (Ravnskov, 2002).

High cholesterol levels are a risk factor, not a causal factor. Risk factors are not diseases, but risk factors have now been turned into diseases.

Before we go any further, we should first define what high cholesterol is. Over the years, the definition of "high cholesterol" has been revised on a regular basis. It seems that the cut-off point that defines "high cholesterol" is becoming lower, and lower, so that more and more healthy people are being put into the abnormal category and therefore need "treatment".

Who makes these definitions?

Usually, a consensus committee has a meeting and decides on the newer guidelines. In the 2004 revision of what constitutes "high cholesterol", eight out of the nine experts were paid consultants to big pharmaceutical companies, which just happened to make cholesterol lowering drugs.

Perhaps a conflict of interest?

So, I ask again, does a high serum cholesterol level cause heart disease? Or is high serum cholesterol a marker of some underlying metabolic problem that raises cholesterol and causes heart disease at the same time?

Let's return to the basic theme of this book. Our western diet is terrible, high in sugars and refined carbohydrates and TFAs. This diet leads to a metabolic condition known as hyperinsulinaemia: that is, high insulin levels in the blood. I have referred to this numerous times in the book.

It is the sugars and refined carbohydrates in the diet that raise the cholesterol, not the cholesterol in the diet. This high carbohydrate diet stimulates insulin which also encourages the formation of cholesterol.

The hallmark of heart disease is atherosclerosis, the clogging up of the arteries. This clogging up impedes blood flow which can lead to heart attacks and strokes.

Experiments performed by Cruz, Amatuzio, Grande, and Hay (1961) showed the effect of insulin on arteries. In the experiment, insulin was injected into one leg artery of an experimentally induced diabetic dog and placebo (saline) was injected into the artery of the other leg. This was done daily for eight months. When the arteries were examined, the artery that had insulin injected had quite severe atherosclerosis while the saline side was normal. This would indicate that it is the high insulin levels, the hyperinsulinaemia, that can cause the arteries to clog up.

Lowering cholesterol levels *per se* will not necessarily reduce heart disease.

It is interesting to note that, under the age of 50, there seems to be some association between raised cholesterol levels and heart disease, but over the age of 65, this association begins to disappear. In fact, over the age of 75, the higher the levels of cholesterol, the higher the life expectancy (Beckett, Nunes, & Bulpitt, 2000).

Krumholz et al. (1994) showed no association between cholesterol and coronary heart disease mortality and morbidity and all-cause mortality in persons older than 70 years.

Low cholesterol levels in the 71-93 age group showed increased mortality (Schatz et al., 2001).

In 1997, Weverling-Rijnsburger et al. wrote *"In people older than 85 years, high total cholesterol concentrations are associated with longevity owing to lower mortality from cancer and infection."*

Liang, Vetrano, and Qiu (2017) showed that *"The inverse association between high total cholesterol and reduced all-cause mortality in older adults is primarily due to non-cardiovascular mortality..."*

There is another possibility.

Malhotra, Redberg, and Meier (2017) write that coronary heart disease is not caused by saturated fat but is caused by an inflammatory condition.

Henein, Vancheri, Longo, and Vancheri (2022) concluded that *"Atherosclerosis is a chronic inflammatory disease, in which the immune system has a prominent role in its development and progression. Inflammation-induced endothelial dysfunction results in an increased permeability to lipoproteins and their subendothelial accumulation, leukocyte recruitment, and platelets activation."*

If the underlying mechanism is inflammation, it follows that anti-inflammatory agents could reduce inflammation and therefore protect against heart disease.

Li et al. (2020), Cox et al. (2020) and Singh, Sharma, Xu, Tewari, and Fang (2021) showed that curcumin, an extract of turmeric (*Curcumin longa*), an anti-inflammatory herb, can prevent and treat cardiovascular disease.

The herb, hawthorn (*Crataegus spp)* has been used for a long time to treat heart disease. Crataegus has antioxidant, positive inotropic, anti-inflammatory, anti-cardiac remodelling, antiplatelet aggregation, vasodilating, and endothelial protective effects. It is also beneficial in smooth muscle cell migration and proliferation-reduction, ischemia/reperfusion injury protection, lipid-lowering, decreasing arterial blood pressure, and as an antiarrhythmic herb (Alp, Soner, Baysal, & Şahin, 2015).

Khan et al. (2021) concluded that "*Omega-3 FAs reduced cardiovascular mortality and improved cardiovascular outcomes. The cardiovascular risk reduction was more prominent with EPA monotherapy than with EPA+DHA.*"

Omega 3 is known for its anti-inflammatory action.

Another useful herb is ashwagandha (*Withania somnifera*), which is very useful as an adaptogen, to help the body deal with stress. Stress can lead to heart disease. This herb can increase energy and assist with sleep. This seems paradoxical: the herb acts as a cortisol modulator. Modulating cortisol levels can also be beneficial in addressing heart health. Ashwagandha also has an anti-inflammatory action (KrishnaRaju, Somepalli, Thanawala, & Shah, 2023).

Another option is the use of medicinal cannabis (MC). MC has a prominent anti-inflammation activity. This will be discussed later.

Where does this inflammation come from? Esposito and Giugliano (2004) showed that inflammation is a part of MetS.

Insulin is anti-inflammatory (Dandona, Chaudhuri, Mohanty, & Ghanim, 2007) but when there is IR, it becomes pro-inflammatory (Dandona, Aljada, & Bandyopadhyay, 2004).

In summary, MetS produces inflammation in the endothelium producing an endothelial dysfunction which then produces artery disease which leads to cardiovascular disease. The use of natural anti-inflammatories, such as curcumin, omega 3 oils, or MC, can treat, prevent and/or reduce cardiovascular disease.

A diet full of anti-inflammatory foods such as olive oil, fish, dark green leafy vegetables, berries, dark chocolate (low sugar, low dairy), walnuts, almonds, tomatoes, avocados, colourful vegetables, curries (contains turmeric), ginger, cayenne pepper, and red capsicum can be very helpful in preventing heart disease.

Conversely, pro-inflammatory foods should be avoided. These include sugar, fried foods, refined carbohydrates, alcohol, and meat cooked at high temperatures. Meat cooked at lower temperatures, e.g., slow cooked, or fast cooking e.g., stir fried has a reduced amount of advanced glycation end-products (AGE) which can act as pro-inflammatory agents.

From this, hopefully you can appreciate the basis of a healthy diet.

Statins

We cannot have a chapter on cholesterol without discussing *statins.*

Statins are drugs that are designed to lower cholesterol, and they do lower cholesterol. However, the question to ask is *"does a lower cholesterol prevent heart disease?"*

We have seen so far that it possibly does not.

Mainstream doctors have been pushing statin drugs, especially since the risk factor "high cholesterol" was converted into a disease, and the definition of "high cholesterol" was broadened to include a large majority of the population.

Just one brand (no names mentioned) is a $10

billion a year cash cow for the drug company.

The first statin was extracted from a fungus, *Monascus purpurus* or otherwise known as red yeast rice (RYR) which has been used in Asian cooking and medicine for a very long time. The first statin, lovastatin (commercially known as Mevacor) was a direct extract of the fungus (therefore can be considered a mycotoxin). Recently the pharmaceutical company that makes lovastatin had the audacity to try and ban RYR, because it "contains their drug."

Other companies soon joined in and released their own form of ~~mycotoxin~~ statins.

RYR has been shown to reduce mortality, major cardiovascular events, and risk factors for MetS (Yuan et al., 2022; Sungthong, Yoothaekool, Promphamorn, & Phimarn, 2020).

This is the problem when drug companies extract one component ("the active component") from a herb or some other natural product. The "drug" may not be as good or safe as the whole natural product, as it is missing all the "checks and balances" that are found in the whole mixture.

I will repeat the question; *"Does lowering cholesterol with a drug improve health and/or reduce heart attacks?"*

This is debatable.

There have been many studies where a statin is compared to a placebo and the results look good.

The first major study, the **S**candinavian **S**imvastatin **S**urvival **S**tudy (otherwise known as the 4S study) claimed a 29% reduction in deaths. This is a very impressive figure, but we must look at this carefully. We must distinguish between "relative" and "absolute" figures. In the 4S study, 111 (5%) died of heart attack in the drug group and 189 (8.5%) died in the placebo group. In absolute figures there was only a 3.5% difference: but relative to each other, the difference was 29%. That sounds more impressive.

While it sounds impressive, it would give a totally wrong impression.

The 4S study had other problems, there were no women, no elderly, no children, yet statins are given to all these groups.

Newer studies have been done, again, expressing the results as relative figures.

It is important to note that relative figures are used to give the appearance of a better outcome, i.e. to make the drug look better, yet side effects are given in absolute terms to give the appearance of making it look safer.

Diamond and Leaverton (2023) wrote that *"The manner in which clinical trial investigators present their findings to healthcare providers and the public can have a substantial influence on their impact. For example, if a heart attack occurs in 2% of those in the placebo group and in 1% of those in the drug-treated group, the benefit to the treated population is only one percentage point better than no treatment. This finding is unlikely to generate much enthusiasm from the study sponsors and in the reporting of the findings to the public. Instead, trial directors can amplify the magnitude of the appearance of the treatment benefit by using the relative risk (RR) value of a 50% reduction of the risk of a heart attack, since one is 50% of two."*

Many other studies have been done, most show benefit but, again, with this statistical fiddle.

The ALLHAT (**A**ntihypertensive and **L**ipid **L**owering Treatment to Prevent **H**eart **A**ttack **T**rial) study which ran from 1994 to 2002**,** used pravastatin in 5,170 participants aged 55 and over and compared them to 5,185 participants on "usual care". The group was a diverse group of people, with a mean age of 66 years, consisting of 49% women, 38% black, 23% Hispanic, 14% had a history of coronary heart disease (CHD) and

35% had T2D. This diverse group probably better reflects the general population than the select group used in previous studies. After four years the cholesterol level was lowered by 17% in the pravastatin group and 8% in the "usual care" group, so "yes" the drug can lower cholesterol. However, after six years there was no significant difference in death from all causes and from CHD between the two groups. (Pasternak, 2002)

As I have already said, lowering the risk factors does not necessarily reduce the risk.

Unfortunately, this ALLHAT study has been virtually buried because it did not show what the all-powerful drug companies wanted to show. The interesting fact is that the ALLHAT study was sponsored by the USA government, not by a drug company.

Figures do not lie BUT you can lie with figures.

A meta-analysis by Byrne et al. (2022) determined *"A conclusive association between absolute reductions in LDL-C levels and individual clinical outcomes was not established...."*

Niacin (vitamin B3) has been shown to reduce

LDL (the "bad" cholesterol) and increase HDL (the "good" cholesterol). This improvement in cholesterol *should* favour improvement in heart morbidity, heart mortality and strokes. However, Schandelmaier et al. (2017) showed that despite the favourable HDL/LDL achieved by niacin, there was no reduction in mortality, cardiovascular mortality, non-cardiovascular mortality, the number of fatal and non-fatal heart attacks, nor the number of fatal or non-fatal strokes.

Niacin produces favourable changes in cholesterol levels but does not influence heart attacks, strokes, or mortality.

So, is it really the cholesterol that is causing heart disease? Is it really the cholesterol lowering ability of statins that produce the benefit?

How can we tie all this together?

Rosenson and Tangney (1998) raised the point that statins have effects other than lowering cholesterol: this is why they can have an effect in situations where cholesterol is not an issue. They concluded that *"baseline or treated LDL cholesterol levels are only weakly associated with net coronary angiographic change or cardiovascular events."* They suggested that the benefits of statins are due to "*a non-cholesterol lowering mechanism that modifies endothelial function, inflammatory responses, plaque stability and thrombus formation."*

This property of statins is called the *pleiotropic effect*. This includes anti-inflammatory effects, antioxidant effects, antiproliferative and immunomodulatory effects, plaque stability, normalisation of sympathetic outflow, and prevention of platelet aggregation (Kavalipati, Shah, Ramakrishan, & Vasnawala, 2015).

So, the question must be asked; is it the cholesterol lowering effect that protects against heart disease, or is it the pleiotropic effect? We have already seen that improving cholesterol levels does not necessarily improve heart morbidity and mortality, except possibly in the under 50 age group.

There is a new category of drugs, still experimental, called cholesteryl ester transfer protein inhibitors (CETP inhibitors), such as evacetrapib, torcetrapib, anacetrapib, and dalcetrapib. These drugs have been shown to increase HDL (the "good" cholesterol) and reduce the LDL (the "bad" cholesterol) – so these drugs *should* prevent heart disease because they produce "favourable" cholesterol levels.

However, they do not protect against heart disease: from this we can possibly conclude that cholesterol levels are not the main cause of heart disease.

Menon et al. (2020) studied the effects of a CETP inhibitor in patients with T2D. The researchers concluded that *"Despite a favorable increase in HDL and decreases in LDL and HbA1c levels in patients with DM, we observed no benefits of treatment with evacetrapib on prespecified clinical outcomes in this high-risk population."*

In another study looking at CTEP inhibitors in high-risk vascular disease, Lincoff et al. (2017) concluded *"Although the cholesteryl ester transfer protein inhibitor evacetrapib had favorable effects on established lipid biomarkers, treatment with evacetrapib did not result in a lower rate of cardiovascular events than placebo among patients with high-risk vascular disease."*

So, I ask again: is it the pleiotropic effects of the statins that produce the effects? It certainly does not seem to be the cholesterol reducing effects *per se*.

All you hear from the mainstream is that high cholesterol levels are dangerous and are sure to kill you, but as we discussed earlier:

- cholesterol is not a factor in the elderly: high

cholesterol level can be a sign of longevity.

- Petursson, Sigurdsson, Bengtsson, Nilsen, and Getz (2012) stated that elevated cholesterol in women may prove to be not only harmless but even beneficial.
- I would say that it is obvious that statins are not needed where there are "normal" levels of cholesterol.

Statins are not needed in the elderly, for women, or for normal levels.

This brings us to the next point.

Can heart disease be prevented by giving statins? This is called primary prevention. Can we prevent future heart disease by giving a statin to normal people? Drug companies would like this; there are dollar ign in their eye$.

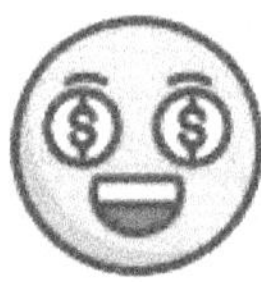

Put everyone on statins and prevent heart disease. There is even a suggestion (hopefully tongue in cheek) of putting statins into the water supply!

In the Therapeutic Letter (April-May-June 2003) published by the University of British Colombia, the researchers concluded,

"Therefore, statins have not been shown to provide an overall health benefit in primary prevention trials." (*www.ti.ubc.ca/PDF/48.pdf* - Accessed 25 August 2023)

Redburg and Katz (2017) wrote that the data is weak for the use of statins as primary prevention in asymptomatic patients.

In a study of twelve European countries, there was no statistical change between coronary heart disease (CHD) and statin use, nor between changes in CHD and changes in statin use between 2000 and 2012 (Vancheri, Backlund, Strender, Godman, & Wettermark, 2016).

In summary, statins have been shown to work only in men under age 50 and even then, the results are modest and does not necessarily have anything to do with cholesterol lowering *per se.*

So, all those women and elderly on statins … do they really need to take them?

Walsh and Pignone (2004) showed that primary prevention in women, i.e. reducing cholesterol in women who do not have cardiovascular disease, does not lower total or coronary heart disease (CHD) mortality. They also showed that in secondary prevention, treatment of hyperlipidaemia reduces CHD events, CHD mortality, non-fatal heart attacks and revascularisation but it <u>does</u>

not affect total mortality. This means that lowering lipids may prevent you from dying of heart disease but does not seem to protect you from dying of some other cause.

An editorial in *JAMA Internal Medicine*, Habib, Katz, and Redberg (2022) questioned the benefit of primary prevention with the use of statins.

As with any drug, not only should we look at the positive side, even though it may be modest, but we should also look at the negative side. Also consider that statins used for primary prevention need to be taken for prolonged periods and starting at an early age.

All drugs have side effects; and statins are no exception.

> *"If it doesn't have side effects, it is not a drug."*

There is a long list of side effects that can occur. These include:

- Nausea
- Diabetes
- Irritability and short tempers
- Hostility

- Homicidal impulses
- Rapid loss of mental capacity
- Amnesia
- Kidney failure
- Diarrhoea
- Muscle aching and weakness
- Tingling or cramping in the legs
- Inability to walk
- Problems sleeping
- Constipation
- Impaired muscle formation
- Erectile dysfunction
- Temperature regulation problems
- Nerve damage
- Mental confusion
- Liver damage and abnormalities
- Neuropathy
- Destruction of Coenzyme Q10, a vital nutrient.
- Cancer

Many drugs have long lists of side effects and the important thing to know is the incidence of these side effects. How common are they? How rare are they?

A meta-analysis by Bytyçi et al. (2022) showed a side effect (or as they called it statin intolerance) incidence of 9.1%.

However, in an on-line survey by Radar Television in the Netherlands in 2006, those on statins reported a 27.1% incidence of side effects. A study/survey like this may not be scientific and can be criticized (and has been) but 27.1% of people complaining of side effects is a significant number.

(https://spacedoc.com › articles › the-netherlands-radar-survey - Accessed 25 August 2023)

Sheldon (2007) criticized the TV programme. *"The programme,* Radar, *broadcast by television company Televisie Radio Omroep Stichting, also raised doubts about the safety of prescribing statins to combat high cholesterol. Doctors fear that some of the one million Dutch patients who are taking statins may stop without consulting their doctor and, therefore, risk future heart attacks."*

The doctors are blaming the TV programme for highlighting the fact that there are side effects of statins and blaming patients for wanting to stop the medication.

Just under 50% of patients prescribed statins for primary prevention stop taking the medication. For secondary prevention 41% stop. However, 72% of primary prevention, and 75% of secondary prevention patients, do re-start (Vinogradova, Coupland, Brindle, & Hippisley-Cox, 2016).

Is this because of "medical gaslighting"?

The mainstream lament that many people stop the statins because of side effects and try hard to dismiss the patient's concerns.

Studies show a similar incidence of side effects in the placebo group as in the statin group. So why do many complain of side effects? Is it just the thought of taking a pill, especially a statin?

There has been a lot of talk about statins on social media and perhaps people are influenced by this.

Many patients who are rechallenged can tolerate the statins long-term (Zhang et al., 2013).

Many doctors claim that these side effects such as muscle pains are "in your head". Though remember that pain is pain no matter what the cause.

Other doctors encourage patients to "push through" the side effects because the medication is there to protect you from heart disease; *"It's for your own good!"*

I could call this "medical gaslighting"!

Statin side effects

A significant side effect of statins is the development of T2D (Culver et al., 2012). However, this increase is mainly in the elderly, who have other diabetes risk factors and are on a high dose (Mansi, Sumithran, & Kinaan, 2023).

However, I must point out that if there is high cholesterol, then there is a chance that the person has MetS, which makes it more likely that T2D can develop.

In the Veteran Affairs Diabetes Trial (VADT), military veterans with T2D were followed and showed that the veterans who were using statins more frequently showed greater progression of vascular calcification compared with diabetic veterans who were using statins less frequently (Saremi, Bahn, Reaven; VADT Investigators., 2012).

Mansi et al. (2021) showed that statin use was associated with diabetes progression, and a greater chance of needing insulin injections and a greater chance of needing diabetes medications, with also an increased likelihood of diabetic complications.

Cederberg et al. (2016) concluded *'Statin treatment increased the risk of type 2 diabetes by 46%, attributable to decreases in insulin sensitivity and insulin secretion."*

Statins not only block the synthesis of cholesterol but also block the biosynthesis of coenzyme Q10 (CoQ10), a very important nutrient that is an essential component of mitochondria, the energy producing units of the cells. CoQ10 is critical in the production of energy. Without CoQ10, there is no energy: the cell is like a car without the spark plugs.

Giving statins to patients with congestive cardiac failure (CCF) has been shown to reduce the already low level of CoQ10 and aggravate the heart failure. Patients with CCF should not be given statins, or alternatively, should be supplemented with CoQ10 (Langsjoen & Langsjoen, 2003; Folkers et al., 1990).

More recently, Niazi, Galehdar, Jamshidi, Mohammadi, and Moayyedkazemi (2020) wrote *"Recently, it has been hypothesized that, despite the positive effects reported, high doses of statins in patients with long-term heart failure leads to progress in heart failure by inhibiting CoQ10 synthesis and intensifying hypertrophy..."*

This reduction of CoQ10 is possibly also the same cause for the common side effect of muscle weakness and muscle aches. (Don't forget that the heart is a muscle as well.) It is found that supplementing CoQ10 can reduce many of these muscle side effects.

Why aren't the drug companies releasing this information?

This is not to say that they have not thought about it.

One of the world's largest pharmaceutical companies, Merck & Co, took out a US Patent in 1990, on a capsule, combining CoQ10 with a statin.

(https://patents.google.com/patent/US4933165A/en. - Accessed 26 August 2023)

The company must have known that there may be problems or else they would not have done this.

Okuyama et al. (2015) rejected the current belief that statins decrease atherosclerosis and discussed that statins may be a *cause* of coronary calcification. Statins are mitochondrial toxins (statins were first extracted from a fungus and as such are a mycotoxin) that impair the muscular function of the heart by depleting CoQ10, and therefore reducing adenosine triphosphate (ATP) generation in the heart and blood vessels. ATP is the organic compound that provides energy to drive and support many processes in living cells.

Statins inhibit the biosynthesis of seleno-proteins, notably glutathione peroxidase, which is an important antioxidant and the body's main detoxifier. This can also be a factor in the development of congestive cardiac failure (CCF), similar to cardiomyopathies related to selenium deficiency.

Statins also inhibit the synthesis and functionality of vitamin K2, which therefore interferes with its role of protecting arteries from calcification.

Vitamin K

There are 2 major forms of vitamin K – vitamin K1 (phylloquinone) mainly plant based and vitamin K2 (menaquinone) which comes mainly from fermented products (natto, sauerkraut, kefir, Greek yoghurt, apple cider vinegar), animal sources (meat, liver, egg yolks, hard cheese) and can also be made by the gut microbiota (Yan et al., 2022).

Vitamin K1 can be converted to vitamin K2.

Natto, the Japanese fermented soybean, is probably one of the highest sources of vitamin K2.

Vitamin K is a fat-soluble vitamin, therefore needs fat for optimal absorption. Vitamin K2 is the more active form in bone building and prevention of calcium depositing into arteries. A lack of vitamin K2 can aggravate calcium deposits into arteries. As noted above, statins interfere with vitamin K2 action. In a study by Zhelyazkova-Savova et al. (2021), the researchers compared statin users who had established cardiovascular disease with non-statin users who were healthy who had a moderate cardiovascular risk. They found statin users had lower vitamin K2 dependent proteins and higher levels of vascular calcification. This ties in with the Veteran Affairs Diabetes Trial as discussed above.

Ironically, vitamin K2 is in foods we have been told not to eat such as eggs, fat, and meat because of "heart health". Vitamin K is virtually non-existent in "junk food", leading to vitamin K2 deficiency which impairs the calcium removal and increases risk of blood vessel calcification (Maresz, 2015).

Cholesterol is an essential nutrient; it is the starting point for all our steroid hormones, vitamin D, and the basic building blocks of all our cell membranes; a large percentage of our brain is cholesterol.

Can low cholesterol, either naturally or produced by statins, influence our brains or our hormones?

Yes, it can.

Lovastatin (one of the statins) has been shown to reduce performance on neuropsychological testing of attention and psychomotor speed (Muldoon et al., 2000).

Low cholesterol can cause aggressive behaviour and depression (Hillbrand, Waite, Miller, Spitz, & Lingswiler, 2000).

Low cholesterol is related to depression in men (Steegmans, Hoes, Bak, van der Does, & Grobbee, 2000) and women (Horsten, Wamala, Vingerhoets, & Orth-Gomer,1997).

Low cholesterol is associated with increased criminal violence (Golomb, Stattin, & Mednick, 2000).

Low serum total cholesterol level is associated with an increased risk of suicide (Ellison, & Morrison, 2001).

Low cholesterol can be considered as a biological marker for risk of suicide in depressed patients (Kim & Myint, 2004).

However, newer studies (Parsaik et al., 2014; De Giorgi et al., 2021) suggested that statin use is associated with a lower risk of depression.

Is it the low cholesterol *per se* or is it the low cholesterol produced by taking statins, or is it the statins itself that is causing the problems?

Impotence and reduced libido have been attributed to statins. *"Decreased libido is a probable adverse drug* *reaction of HMG-CoA-reductase-inhibitors (*statins*) and is reversible. The ADR (*Adverse Drug Reaction*) may be caused by low serum testosterone levels, mainly due to intracellular cholesterol depletion"* (de Graaf, Brouwers, & Diemont, 2004).

*"Multivariate analysis showed that erectile dysfunction was dependant on treatment with fibrate (*another cholesterol lowering medication*) derivative….and statins"* (Bruckert, Giral, Heshmati, & Turpin,1996).

Erectile difficulties can be considered a sensitive indicator of the state of the arteries in general and are considered a good marker of pre-morbid heart disease (Billups, Bank, Padma-Nathan, Katz, & Williams, 2005).

So, men, if you have good erections, then your blood vessels are in a good condition, not just in the penis but also your heart.

However, newer studies show that statins may improve erectile dysfunction because of the vascular effects of the statins (Kostis & Dobrzynski, 2019).

Could these side effects be due to low cholesterol (not specifically to statin use.) Statins can reduce cholesterol too low. Sahebzamani et al. (2013) showed a relationship between low cholesterol and depressive symptoms, aggression, hostility, and cynicism.

Low cholesterol levels have also been shown to be associated with violent crime (Golomb, Stattin, & Mednick 2000).

Who do we believe? Studies are known to be chosen and paid for by pharmaceutical companies to highlight their products, also to bury any negative studies. Also well known is that some companies will fund new research just to counter any earlier studies that discredit them. It is interesting to note that the newer studies on statins have opposite results to that of earlier studies.

See *When big companies fund academic research, the truth often comes last.*

(https://www.sydney.edu.au › news-opinion › news › 2019 › 10 › 03 › when-big-companies-fund-academic-research - Accessed 26 Aug 2023)

See also Ioannidis (2017) "*Why most published research findings are false.*"

Of course, we must not lose sight of the fact that there are a lot of people (and the number is increasing) in western society that have blocked, atherosclerotic arteries. This is most likely caused by the underlying metabolism that I have constantly referred to in this book. This is due to the hyperinsulinaemia caused by the high carbohydrate western diet.

Researchers from the University of California have shown that statins (simvastatin, pravastatin) are cancer producing. A review by Newman and Hulley (1996) showed that statins stimulate cancer in rats.

Humans are not rodents, and the results of animal experiments cannot be directly correlated to humans, but this result should have had some bearing on the eventual approval of this drug for human use. The excuse was that the doses used in animals were very much higher than in humans. However, if the blood levels are considered, then the animal models achieve very similar blood levels as human patients.

Statins stimulate vascular endothelial growth factor (VEGF). They share a similar pathway, and statins have been shown to activate angiogenesis, i.e. stimulates new blood vessel growth. This may be beneficial to revascularize heart muscle after a heart attack, but is a worry because angiogenesis is also an important factor in the development of cancerous growths (Skaletz-Rorowski & Walsh, 2003).

In the CARE (**C**holesterol **A**nd **R**ecurrent **E**vents) study, breast cancer was more common in the drug group than the placebo group. It was explained away as an "anomaly".

Unfortunately, time will tell whether it was an anomaly or not, but by then, unfortunately, it will be too late for many who do develop cancer.

Chang, Ho, Chiu, and Yang (2011) showed that statins increase the risk of prostate cancer.

Newer studies are now showing that statins may actually be used to improve survivability in cancer (Yang et al., 2020; Fatehi Hassanabad, 2019).

A 2011 study by Vinogradova, Coupland, and Hippisley-Cox, showed that statins were not associated with increased cancer risk at the most common sites, except for colorectal, bladder and lung cancers. There was a reduced risk of haematological cancers.

In an editorial (Goldstein, Mascitelli, & Pezzetta, 2008), the authors concluded that there was *"ample evidence that statins may promote cancer in certain segments of the population."*

So, which is it? Do statins cause cancer, or can they be used to treat it?

Remember that statin usage is long term.

Statins may cause liver damage, so it is advisable

that all patients on any of the statins have regular liver checks.

Does the use of statins out-weigh the risk? Are statins as good as they say?

Kristensen, Christensen, and Hallas (2015) concluded that *"Statin treatment results in a surprisingly small average gain in overall survival within the trials' running time. For patients whose life expectancy is limited or who have adverse effects of treatment, withholding statin therapy should be considered."*

So, what can we do to protect ourselves?

Since the major cause of elevated cholesterol is IR, all efforts should be aimed at dealing with the underlying MetS, which is the main theme of this book.

So, do we treat high cholesterol?

There are many who are so paranoid, so totally fearful of the dogma that cholesterol is dangerous that they insist on being treated with statins.

On the other hand, there are those who are so totally fearful of statins that they refuse to be treated with them. For these people, diet and lifestyle advice are a must.

Using statins alone will lower cholesterol but will it protect against heart disease? Statins can be used in conjunction with making lifestyle changes, nutrition changes, and using supplements. If the cholesterol does come down, the statins can be stopped, however, monitoring should continue.

Summary

Cholesterol is a very important molecule for the body and has many roles. It is a major building block for the cell membranes and for the intracellular organelles. The cells need the waxy properties of cholesterol to keep the cell framework intact, as well as to keep the flow of molecules into and out of the cell.

It is the starting molecule for the synthesis of vitamin D, all steroid hormones and sex hormones.

Cholesterol is a main component of the bile acids which are needed for proper digestion of foods, especially fats, and for absorption of the fat-soluble vitamins, A, D and E. Cholesterol is important for the growth of brain and nervous tissue. Since it is a part of the cell structure it is needed for cellular repair.

As you can see, cholesterol is an essential nutrient for humans. It really does not deserve the bad publicity it gets. Up till recently, high cholesterol levels were regarded as bad, and the emphasis was to lower it as much as possible. That is, the lower the better. This is not necessarily a good thing.

Too low a cholesterol level can be dangerous. This is evidenced by the fact that medical problems seem to occur with a very low serum cholesterol. We have already seen that in the elderly, a low serum cholesterol is a predictor of earlier death.

Some of the studies of cholesterol lowering drugs showed an increased death rate due to non-cardiac reasons in those with a low cholesterol level. So, we may get some protection from heart disease, but we die of something else.

What is the point? The only difference is the diagnosis on the death certificate!

Perhaps the most important factor is the amount of carbohydrate in the diet, especially sugar, the grains, and dairy, as well as other "bad" food factors such as TFAs.

Our nutrition and diet determine how much cholesterol the liver makes.

The biggest problem is that the average person

wants to continue their current diet and lifestyle. They want to continue to consume the white bread, soft drinks, potato wedges, chips, cakes, sugary foods, beer, etc. and still want to remain healthy ... or at least have lower cholesterol.

The "one pill a day and all is well" mentality is an attitude that promotes laziness. Health depends on working on an optimal diet and lifestyle. True health is earned, not provided by a pill.

"Leave your drugs in the chemist's pot if you can heal the patient with food."
Hippocrates (c460 – c370 BCE)

HYPERTENSION

"The good physician treats the disease; the great physician treats the patient who has the disease."
William Osler (1849 – 1919)

Hypertension (and closely related, heart disease) is the fourth component of the "deadly quartet". We have already looked at the three other components and have seen that there are similarities. They are not necessarily diseases, but they are all symptoms. They are just numbers, and they are superficial manifestations of an underlying metabolic issue. It is important to deal with the underlying metabolism, and as we shall see, simply lowering the numbers will not necessarily produce better health.

High blood pressure (BP) may not cause heart disease … What!? … high BP is a symptom of heart and artery disease; and as we have seen earlier, just treating the symptoms may not improve health: though there is an exception that we shall see later.

The largest category of hypertension (92-94%) is called "essential hypertension" which is where, up till recently, no cause could be found. There are rarer types of high BP (e.g., endocrine, renal artery stenosis, aortic coarctation) which, when the cause is found and fixed, the high BP is cured.

Essential hypertension is more than likely caused by the disturbed underlying metabolism that I have been discussing so far in this book. Reaven and Hoffman (1989) showed that hypertensive patients were hyperinsulinaemic when compared to normal controls.

High BP is largely a problem of the arteries. Any arterial narrowing or stiffness causes the heart to beat stronger and with a higher pressure just to keep the blood circulating; this is a reflex compensatory mechanism to ensure continuing blood flow.

If the arteries narrow more, or become stiffer, the blood pressure goes up. The heart muscle bulks up, like Arnold Schwarzenegger, which again is a compensatory mechanism. Initially the enlarged heart muscle beats stronger and efficiently but beyond a crucial point the excessively enlarged heart muscle becomes inefficient and heart failure could develop.

When the narrowing gets beyond a critical point, then no matter how high the BP is, blood will not flow to various areas, this would lead to heart attacks, strokes, etc.

The problem is with the arteries.

So, the important question to ask is: *"What causes damage to the arteries?"*

We discussed the experiments of Cruz, Amatuzio, Grande, and Hay (1961). They found one major cause of arterial disease is insulin.

The inflammation caused by MetS is another cause of arterial damage.

Another common cause is the multitude of pollutants and chemicals from smoking and from just breathing the air, eating the food, and drinking the water on this contaminated planet of ours.

Other major issues are stress, lack of exercise, lack of sleep and vitamin D deficiency which is epidemic in today's modern society.

Endothelial dysfunction

The first finding of any arterial abnormality is in the endothelium, the inner lining of the arteries and is referred to as *endothelial dysfunction*. As discussed earlier, the endothelium is very resistant to becoming insulin resistant, therefore responds to the elevated levels of insulin.

In 2003, Caballero wrote that *"Obesity, insulin resistance, and endothelial dysfunction closely coexist throughout the natural history of type 2 diabetes. They all can be identified not only in people with type 2 diabetes, but also in various groups at risk for the disease, such as individuals with impaired glucose tolerance, family history of type 2 diabetes, hypertension, dyslipidemia, prior gestational diabetes, or polycystic ovary syndrome."* He also stated that *"Insulin resistance leads to endothelial dysfunction through the frequent association with traditional cardiovascular risk factors and through some more direct novel mechanisms."*

Medina-Leyte et al. (2021) showed that endothelial dysfunction is one of the main causes of atherosclerosis. *"Endothelial dysfunction plays an essential role in the development of atherosclerosis and can be triggered and exacerbated by different cardiovascular and cardiometabolic risk factors."*

The condition of the endothelium is probably the most important factor in the development of artery disease: atherosclerosis, which is possibly the number one major disease of civilization.

Endothelial dysfunction can be regarded as an early stage in the atherosclerotic process and the key that begins the process is IR and the associated inflammation.

IR can cause inflammation, but inflammation can cause the IR. They are associated, they can cause each other, and both can cause endothelial dysfunction.

"A chronic state of inflammation appears to be a central mechanism underlying the pathophysiology of insulin resistance and MetS" (Welty, Alfaddagh, & Elajami, 2016).

Endothelial dysfunction can start very early in life, perhaps even in the foetal stage. We do know that a foetus growing in an elevated insulin environment (e.g., an obese mother) is already set for problems with obesity and high BP, i.e. MetS.

IR and inflammation cause endothelial dysfunction.

Treating and relieving IR and addressing inflammation improves endothelial dysfunction.

Insulin resistance is a key factor in the development of endothelial dysfunction.

"Metabolic insulin resistance is characterized by pathway-specific impairment in phosphatidylinositol 3-kinase dependant signalling, which in endothelium may cause imbalance between production of NO (nitric oxide) and secretion of endothelin-1 leading to decreased blood flow, which worsens insulin resistance" (Kim, Montagnani, Koh, & Quon, 2006).

"Insulin resistance and Endothelial Dysfunction play a central role in the pathogenesis of atherosclerosis. Much evidence supports the presence of insulin resistance as the fundamental pathophysiologic disturbance responsible for the cluster of metabolic and cardiovascular disorders, known collectively as the metabolic syndrome. Endothelial dysfunction is an important component of the metabolic or insulin resistance syndrome and this is demonstrated by inadequate vasodilation and/or paradoxical vasoconstriction in coronary and peripheral arteries in response to stimuli that release nitric oxide (NO)" (Cersosimo & DeFronzo, 2006).

Our western diet is a major cause of the development of IR and inflammation. This is the starting point of all our troubles.

Smoke and pollution

Other causes of endothelial dysfunction are chemicals and pollutants. Perhaps the most common form of pollution is self-pollution, caused by smoking. Zeiher, Schächinger, and Minners (1995) demonstrated that chemicals from cigarettes are absorbed and cause arterial damage.

Even passive smokers are not safe. Passive smoke can damage arteries almost as much as active smoking. The good news is that it may be reversible, to a certain extent, although this depends heavily on the amount and length of exposure (Raitakari, Adams, McCredie, Griffiths, & Celermajer, 1999).

Here again, the initial damage is endothelial dysfunction.

We live on a polluted planet. We breathe in polluted air every day, and this can damage our arteries. If you live on a main road, there are plenty of diesel fumes that can be breathed in. Törnqvist et al. (2007) showed that *"... combustion-derived air pollution may have an important systemic and adverse vascular effects for at least 24 hours following exposure."*

If a single exposure produces effects for 24 hours, what will happen with continual exposure?

Heavy metals

Other pollutants in this toxic world of ours are the heavy metals (HMs), such as lead (Pb), mercury (Hg), cadmium (Cd) and arsenic (As). They cause vascular disease by

- Increased oxidative stress,
- Inflammation,
- Disruption of enzyme function.

Hagele et al. (2007) showed that Hg can be a risk factor of cardiovascular disease.

In a systematic review, Navas-Acien, Guallar, Silbergeld, and Rothenberg (2007) demonstrated that HM pollutants, especially Pb, are linked to hypertension.

"Individuals with blood lead levels of 20 to 29 micro g/dL in 1976 to 1980 (15% of the US population at that time) experienced significantly increased all-

cause, circulatory, and cardiovascular mortality from 1976 through 1992" (Lustberg & Silbergeld, 2002).

In 2004, Navas-Acien et al. wrote that *"Blood lead and cadmium, at levels well below current safety standards, were associated with an increased prevalence of peripheral arterial disease in the general US population. Cadmium may partially mediate the effect of smoking on peripheral arterial disease."*

Nash et al. (2003) wrote *"At levels well below the current US occupational exposure limit guidelines (40 µg/dL), blood lead level is positively associated with both systolic and diastolic blood pressure and risks of both systolic and diastolic hypertension among women aged 40 to 59 years. The relationship between blood lead level and systolic and diastolic hypertension is most pronounced in postmenopausal women. These results provide support for continued efforts to reduce lead levels in the general population, especially women."*

One way to treat hypertension is to remove HMs from the body but before HMs can be removed, we must ensure that they are there.

In this polluted world most people will have some degree of HMs poisoning.

Blood tests are useful only in the acute exposure

situation. The body does not like HMs floating in the blood, so, very quickly, the HMs are stored away in the cells. In the chronic situation, blood tests are useless. Urine tests are better. Urine tests pre and post chelation challenge is possibly the gold standard.

The treatment for heavy metal toxicity is chelation (pronounced key-LAY shun) therapy. The word "chelation" comes from the Greek word *"chele"* meaning a claw and refers to the ability of certain molecules to chemically grab onto and hold other molecules. To understand chelation therapy, we must look at a substance called ethylene diamine tetra-acetic acid (EDTA).

EDTA is a synthetic amino acid that was first synthesized by Franz Munz in 1934. It was used in the fabric and textiles industry in Nazi Germany since other chemicals could not be imported due to the political situation.

Later it was shown to form a stable bond with HMs, such as Pb. There were many people poisoned with Pb after WW2, e.g., battery workers and naval personnel who painted ships with lead-based paints. An intravenous infusion of EDTA was found to be safe and effective to remove Pb from the body via the kidneys. That is, EDTA chelated (grabbed) Pb and it then could be urinated out.

Many naval workers were treated with EDTA for Pb poisoning. Coincidentally, it was discovered that many with vascular problems, such as angina and claudication improved significantly. Vascular disease can be treated with chelation therapy, though this is a very controversial issue.

Chelation is the process where an agent, usually EDTA, is introduced into the body, usually intravenously; this agent binds to toxic heavy metals and removes them via the kidneys. For safe chelation, kidney function must be good and therefore, an assessment of kidney function is essential prior to treatment. EDTA infusions can last up to three hours and needs to be done in the clinic environment.

There is another chelating agent called di mercapto succinic acid (DMSA). This can be given orally and is therefore very useful in children and with those where a vein cannot be found. DMSA capsules can be given in the home situation. It is probably the second-best chelating agent.

Stress

The stress of today's modern society adds to the difficulties of maintaining good health. Although not considered in our discussion to a great extent so far, it could possibly be as important an issue as diet with the **diseases of civilization.**

Stress releases cortisol, the adrenal hormone which, in the correct amounts is beneficial and essential, however, too much can cause metabolic derangements. Stress and cortisol are intertwined into this whole problem of MetS.

According to Ghiadoni et al. (2000) even brief episodes of stress, that are normal in everyday life, can cause up to four hours of endothelial dysfunction.

What would happen if the stress was prolonged? What would happen, if at the same time, the person smoked and ate the wrong type of foods, high in sugars and carbohydrates? The combined effect of stress, smoke and insulin would compound the damage.

The stress response, or general adaptive syndrome (GAS) was introduced by the Hungarian Canadian scientist Hans Selye (1907-1982) in 1946. His research led to the discovery that stress can lead to infection, illness, disease, and death. He described three stages: Alarm, Resistance and Exhaustion.

Stage one: Alarm. When the threat or stressor is identified or realised, the body's stress response is a state of alarm. During this stage, adrenaline will be produced to bring a fight or flight response. This prepares the body for life-threatening situations, channelling blood away from the skin, genitals, digestive and immune systems for use in more immediate muscular and emotional needs. This leads to the immune system being depressed, making us susceptible to disease. There is also increased cortisol production.

Stage two: Resistance. If the stressor persists, it becomes necessary to attempt some means of coping with the stress. As we become used to the stress levels, we initially become *more* resistant to disease, which leads us to believe we can easily adapt to these more stressful situations. However, although this is only the immune system fighting to keep up with demands and expectations, the stress requires it to work at abnormally high levels.

Although the body begins to try to adapt to the strains or demands of the environment, it cannot keep this up indefinitely, so its resources are gradually depleted.

Stage three: Exhaustion. In the final stage in the GAS model, all the body's resources are eventually depleted, and the body is unable to maintain normal function. Eventually reality kicks in and our bodies give up on trying to maintain a high level of stress. Parts of the body literally start to break down and we become very unwell. If we continue to fight this situation, we may even die. Some have referred to death as stage four.

At this point the initial symptoms may reappear (sweating, raised heart rate etc.). If stage three is extended, long term damage may result as the capacity of glands, especially the adrenal gland, and the immune system is exhausted, and function is impaired resulting in decompensation. The result can manifest itself in obvious illnesses such as ulcers, cardiovascular problems, and depression, along with other mental issues.

The so-called fight/flight response was developed very early on in our evolution and the survival benefits are easy to see.

Imagine our paleolithic ancestor walking through the forest and coming face to face with a sabre-toothed tiger. The immediate stress response is the secretion of adrenaline, which allowed our ancestors to fight harder and/or run faster! The blood is shunted away from the skin, digestive and sexual organs to the muscles: the blood is needed in the muscles to run and fight. The reduced blood to the skin limits bleeding if injury occurs. Digestion and sex are not a priority while running or fighting. This situation is only a short-term response. More long-term stress is characterized by high cortisol secretion, and this can lead to the long-term effects of stress.

Our society has changed but our adaptive responses have not. We no longer need to run or fight the sabre-toothed tiger.

We live differently now. We work in factories or offices, where running away or fighting is not appropriate and not encouraged. If your boss is always on your back, if there are deadlines to meet, you are stressed, but you cannot run or fight. There are mortgages, bills to be paid, BAS, tax, traffic jams … these are all stressful. We cannot run away. Punching the boss is probably not a good response.

The acute response is the adrenaline secretion. The effects of this manifests as sweating, palpitations, and the feeling of dread. This is interpreted as anxiety. As we have seen, adrenaline shunts blood from the vital organs, such as the digestive system, immune system, and the genitals. It is not hard to see why there is an epidemic of gut problems, sexual problems, and immune system problems.

Modern society imposes many demands, and many people cannot cope. These are the *stressors,* or the causative agents. Stressors can be emotional (demanding job, relationship issues), physical (heat, cold) or mental (pain). Stress is the resulting condition. We do adapt but at what expense? Cortisol levels rise. Cortisol influences the vascular endothelium. Cortisol has other effects: fat accumulation, raising of BSL as well as an aggravation of IR.

Does chronic stress producing high cortisol levels cause MetS?

Is it just the high carbohydrate western diet?

Is it a combination of both?

Is this the reason for the variability of the syndrome?

Stress, or more accurately, cortisol, is a direct cause of endothelial dysfunction.

Here I should point out that cortisol is regarded as anti-inflammatory, but in the chronic situation it can have an opposite effect and become pro-inflammatory (Sorrells, Caso, Munhoz, & Sapolsky, 2009).

Chandola, Brunner, and Marmot (2006) considered that stress is an important risk factor for developing MetS. Their study of 10,308 men and women aged 35-55 found a dose-response relation between work stress and the risk of developing MetS.

Sleep

As we discussed earlier, lack of sleep can cause MetS and therefore can be a factor in hypertension. The modern person is trying to fit more and more into the 24-hour day and as a result is losing sleep. There are, of course, many people, estimated to be about 35% of the population, who have difficulty going to sleep. There are many reasons for this, including anxiety, depression, pain, etc. Poor sleep, snoring and sleep apnoea are symptoms of MetS and can be helped by dietary and life-style changes.

Gangwisch et al. (2006) showed that sleep deprivation, in the short and long term can produce hypertension.

Although not mentioned specifically, exercise, or should I say, a lack of exercise, is also another important factor in the development of hypertension.

The role of exercise should not be underestimated: Pescatello et al. (2004) confirmed that exercise is essential for the primary prevention, treatment, and control of hypertension.

All in all, these factors: i.e. hyperinsulinaemia, pollution, stress, sleep deprivation and (lack of) exercise are all a result of our present western lifestyle and diet and so are causes of the **diseases of civilization.**

We have discussed how insulin sensitivity starts at conception. The health and lifestyle of the mother are a great determinant on the health on the health of the baby. Pregnant women need to take extra care.

Unfortunately, many pregnant women are not looking after themselves. They smoke, drink, take drugs, get stressed, eat a diet high in sugars and carbohydrates, and put on excess weight.

What happens to the foetus if the mother is obese, stressed, and smokes and drinks? This is leading to breeding a generation of unhealthy children, who, in turn, could carry on the trend to the next generation … and the next … This is why, in my introduction, I said that any turn-around would take generations.

Unfortunately, I cannot see any improvement: all I can see is a species that will slowly deteriorate and eventually, extinction is a great probability.

This sounds very pessimistic and hopefully I will be proven wrong.

> *"Illnesses do not come upon us out of the blue. They are developed from small daily sins against Nature. When enough sins have accumulated, illnesses will suddenly appear."*
>
> **Hippocrates (c460-c370 BCE)**

Since BP is relatively easy to measure, all attention is focused on just that. There is an association between heart disease and BP but that does not imply causality. All efforts have been focused on simply lowering BP and as we shall see, the results are not that great.

Up until recently, heart disease has been the number one killer of humans. This has only in the last few years been relegated to the number two spot, being exceeded by deaths from cancer. This doesn't necessarily mean that the incidence of heart disease is reducing, rather it means that fewer people are dying because modern medicine has kept many alive using interventions that have not always been available. However, that people are living longer, does not automatically assume an improvement in health or the quality of life.

So, heart disease and hypertension are big killers, a major category of **Death by Civilization**.

Kaplan described the "Deadly Quartet" in 1989. Reaven and Hoffman (1989) showed that there is a direct relationship between insulin levels and hypertension, as well as showing that IR and high triglycerides are factors that increase the risk of coronary artery disease, and that by reducing or preventing the IR, hypertension can be reduced or prevented.

Further research has shown that hyperinsulinaemia can pre-date hypertension. Therefore, if hyperinsulinaemia can be dealt with early, then hypertension may not develop. This again boils down to diet and life-style changes. The western diet and lifestyle are very favourable to raising insulin levels and therefore to producing MetS.

For many years we have been led to believe that high blood pressure (BP) needs to be reduced to "normal", whatever "normal" is, because high BP causes heart disease. How correct is this?

We have already discussed MetS. We have seen that hypertension is just one of the symptoms. The basic underlying metabolic problem is hyperinsulinaemia: too much insulin in the blood caused by the high carbohydrate western diet.

I have mentioned that simply lowering BP will not necessarily produce better health. You may raise your eyebrows at this considering most doctors are saying that BP needs to be aggressively treated.

To put it into context, lowering extremely high BP can be lifesaving; the high pressure can burst arteries resulting in high morbidity and mortality. However, simply "reducing the numbers" is not enough. The underlying metabolism also needs to be addressed.

Firstly, we must answer the question: "What is normal BP?" It seems that mainstream medicine has drawn an arbitrary line in the sand and anything over that line needs to be treated. This is not specifically correct.

We must define what is high BP. Over the years, the levels have changed. I remember, a long time ago, normal BP was defined as 100 plus your age. "Normal" BP does go up with age. A higher pressure is needed to push blood through the ageing, narrowed, stiff arteries.

Then things changed.

What is considered "normal" has been getting lower and lower. As with cholesterol, the guideline for high BP is decided by a consensus committee and again, as with cholesterol, this consensus committee has a large proportion of doctors who have very close ties with drug companies, who would gain handsomely, if the definition of normal BP levels was changed, i.e. lowered.

The level at which high BP is diagnosed is reducing. This pushes many who were once considered to have normal BP levels into the "abnormal category"; consequently, more and more people will need to be "treated" resulting in increasing numbers of drugs being sold.

A new category of illness has been added to the US guidelines called "pre-hypertension". This is where systolic BP is between 120 and 139 and diastolic between 80 and 89. I would consider these to be normal, especially in older people. Yet people with these readings are now being categorized as "pre-hypertension" and are being treated with medication. For those with "pre-hypertension" the obvious treatment is lifestyle measures, not drugs, however, many are put on drugs, for what is probably an aged dependent normal condition.

Measuring BP is important, although one high reading does not constitute hypertension.

One swallow does not make a summer.

A high reading in the doctor's office can be suspect, the associated stress must be considered. The first stress is simply being at the doctor's surgery.

Are there other factors? Did the person rush to the appointment? Was there a fight with the spouse that morning? Did they just come from the gym after a heavy workout? Did they have a near car crash on the way? Did they just drink a double espresso?

The size of the cuff is also relevant. The right sized cuff must be used. Using a standard sized cuff on a person with a large arm, or *vice versa* will give inaccurate readings. The simple act of having the cuff put onto the arm can raise BP in some. The practitioner should put on the cuff, wait, then measure. If high, remeasure. If the follow up reading is lower, then the BP may be less of a concern. This may not always be achievable, as it takes time and is incompatible with a short consultation.

Factors like these need to be considered.

This elevated BP at the doctor's surgery is referred to as "whitecoat syndrome", or "whitecoat hypertension".

All these factors are important as a one-off high reading in the doctor's office may not necessarily be valid. Home BP monitoring is important. Have the person measure the BP at home, in their own environment. I am more likely to believe the home BP results, rather than the office measurement. However, a high reading at home is significant.

I recently saw a lady whose local doctor frightened her because of a high measurement in the office and wanted to medicate her immediately. Her home BP results were quite normal. She did not need the BP medication that was suggested. I recommended that she continue to monitor her BP and discussed diet and lifestyle changes.

I have also seen people whose BP was high in the doctor's surgery and were put on BP medication. They went home and became unwell, tired, and even fainted from a low BP. These people did not have elevated BP. They simply had a high BP reading in the doctor's surgery.

Does hypertension need to be treated?

Does everyone with a BP beyond that line in the sand need to be treated? There is more to the whole disease than just measuring BP. The problem needs to be looked at wholistically (some spell it holistically). Are there any other factors? Are they elderly? overweight? unfit? smokers? diabetic? Do they have a family history? All these need to be considered. An otherwise fit, healthy, non-smoking, non-diabetic, no family history, elderly man with a BP of 160 may not necessarily need to be treated. All the risk factors need to be considered, realising that risk factors are not the disease and they do not need to be treated as such.

In medical school, we were taught about the risk factors for heart disease. These are hypertension, cholesterol, diabetes, obesity, smoking, ageing, family history, and post-menopausal state. If you look carefully at this list, what can you see? The first four are the symptoms of MetS, the theme of this book. Here again, treatment involves dealing with the underlying metabolism, not just "reducing the numbers".

The initial premise was based on a linear relationship between BP and cardiac mortality i.e. the higher the BP the greater the cardiac death. This is association, not necessarily causation. New modelling does not support this idea. There is a non-linear relationship. Port, Garfinkel, and Boyle (2000) re-analysed the data from the Framingham study and the HOT (Hypertension Optimal Treatment) study and found that this non-linear relationship fitted the data better.

BP does increase with age and therefore that arbitrary line in the sand drawn at 140 mm Hg will put people, especially the elderly, over this line and therefore "needing treatment".

There are lines in the sand, but they are different for different age groups and different for gender.

Port, Garfinkel, and Boyle (2000) showed that this non-linear relationship in the elderly, who have a higher BP, does not necessarily increase risk. Many older people who are on BP medications because their BP is over the line do not necessarily need treatment. Being medicated unnecessarily can lead to a poorer quality of life because of the side effects of these drugs, as well as wasting huge amounts of money on medication, when in many cases, it may not be needed.

MacMahon, Neal, and Rodgers (2005) wrote *"For too long guidelines have supported the belief among doctors and patients that hypertension is a disease...for a vast majority it is not."*

The paper continues that high BP as an isolated finding may not need treatment; other factors need to be considered.

"Although most guidelines acknowledge that such risks are determined by many factors and not by blood pressure alone, this multiplicity of disease determinants is not usually indicated in criteria for the diagnosis or classification of hypertension."

So, what is normal BP?

Or put another way, how low do we have to go to prevent increasing morbidity?

"In the Hypertension Optimal Treatment (HOT) study, hypertensive patients who were randomly assigned to undergo antihypertensive treatment to achieve a goal diastolic blood pressure of 80 mm Hg or lower did not experience fewer cardiovascular events than did patients who received treatment with goal pressures of 85 or 90 mm Hg" (Vidt & Pohl, 1999).

However, in diabetics, this lowering of diastolic BP to 80 mm Hg did result in fewer cardiovascular events. The study also showed that patients on aspirin 75 mg/day had 15% less major cardiovascular events and myocardial infarctions than the placebo group.

There are some doctors who consider that the lower the BP is, the better. There are elderly on multiple medications to get the BP even lower when it may not be necessary.

Does lowering BP produce better health?

We have already seen the results of the MRFIT study, and a similar study done in 1985. In both these studies, BP was lowered to normal but there was little difference in death rates in the treated and non-treated groups.

A long-term study in Sweden looked at hypertensive men and compared them to non-hypertensive men. The two groups were followed for an extended period. The first report (Andersson et al., 1998) was published after following them for over 20 years and another report (Almgren et al., 2005) was published after over 30 years follow up.

These studies showed that hypertensive men, even when the BP is adequately controlled *"... suffered a substantial increased incidence of cardiovascular complications that escalated during the latter course of the study. Their total incidence of stroke was doubled; they had 50% more myocardial infarctions (MIs); mortality from coronary artery disease was increased by a third, compared with non-hypertensive men.*

CONCLUSION: In spite of a substantial reduction of their blood pressure, treated hypertensive middle-aged men had a highly increased risk of stroke, MI and mortality from coronary heart disease compared with non-hypertensive men of similar age."

Just lowering the numbers does not necessarily reduce deaths from heart disease.

It is clear that despite lowering the BP to normal there was still significant morbidity and mortality. Perhaps just "lowering the numbers" isn't enough. Perhaps the underlying metabolism also needs to be addressed.

Risk factors are not diseases, reducing risk factors does not necessarily save lives.

With apologies to Shakespeare *"To treat or not to treat ... that is the question."*

Am I advocating non-treatment of high BP? … No

Am I advocating treating everyone with high BP? … Not necessarily.

Am I advocating looking at the person as a whole, to assess all the factors and also treat the underlying metabolic problem? … Yes.

Excessively high BP (e.g. 180-200+ systolic)

needs to be lowered to prevent cardiovascular damage but at the same time, the underlying metabolism needs to be treated. Once things improve, the medication can be adjusted and possibly even stopped.

It has been said that once medication is started, it cannot be stopped.

I disagree.

If the only treatment was medication, then that would probably be correct. However, if you made lifestyle changes, treated the underlying metabolism, then as the health improved and BP lowered, medication may be reduced and stopped. This does not mean that medication shouldn't be used, even if temporarily while the diet and lifestyle changes are being made. A high BP can cause damage, so a high BP needs to be reduced.

There are even situations where the damage is too far gone and despite all the treatment to the underlying metabolism, the BP doesn't come down. In such a case, medication may need to be continued, albeit at lower doses.

A 62-year-old gentleman was started on a BP medication for high BP by his local doctor. He then saw me for diet and lifestyle advice. About six weeks later I received a frantic call from his wife telling me that he had been dizzy and has fainted on a few occasions. I advised her to check his BP; it was very low. The combination of the BP medication and the dietary and lifestyle advice dropped his BP too low. I suggested he reduce, then possibly stop the BP medication, but advised to continue the lifestyle changes and to continue to monitor the BP.

We have seen that just lowering the numbers does not necessarily give better health. We must look at the underlying metabolism. Here again we are back to the basic theme of the book. Treat the underlying metabolism. Change diet, get more exercise, get more sunshine, stop smoking, use minerals and herbs; and if necessary, start some medication, even if temporarily while waiting for the other measures to start working.

Why did I say, "get more sunshine"?

The human species evolved in the sun. Sunshine is a part of our physiology. An essential nutrient, vitamin D, is made when skin is exposed to sunshine.

Vitamin D has been found to have multiple positive effects on bones, in cancer prevention and on the heart, as well as on many different systems including the immune system.

Vitamin D supplementation has been shown to reduce high BP by improving endothelial dysfunction

(Zittermann, 2003; Carrara et al., 2016), although other studies have shown inconsistent results e.g. Jeong et al. (2017).

One of the most important regulators of BP is the *renin-angiotensin system (RAS).* Angiotensin 2 is a potent vasoconstrictor and anti-natriuretic.

Angiotensin is first produced, by the kidneys, and then is acted upon by renin and *angiotensin converting enzyme (ACE)* to make angiotensin 2.

One of the most popular groups of antihypertensive drugs today is the ACE inhibitor group. These drugs prevent the angiotensin being converted to angiotensin 2. Vitamin D has a similar action. Vitamin D influences the expression of the renin gene and reduces renin activity which also reduces angiotensin being converted to the active angiotensin 2. Vitamin D is a natural ACE inhibitor (Li et al., 2002).

The higher the level of vitamin D, the lower the activity of renin. People living nearer to the equator have less of a problem with high BP compared to people living further north or south, although this study looked at sunlight and temperature, not specifically vitamin D levels; however, vitamin D levels are correlated with sunlight (Cabrera, Mindell, Toledo, Alvo, & Ferro, 2016).

BP is generally higher in the winter as compared to the summer. One of the causes of this elevated BP is vitamin D deficiency. Another reason is the cold weather can cause temporary blood vessel constriction.

Vitamin D also protects against heart attacks. The higher the serum levels of vitamin D, the lower the incidence of heart attacks (Scragg, Jackson, Holdaway, Lim, & Beaglehole,1990).

Why are people vitamin D deficient?

More than likely, it is due to sun paranoia: the fear of the sun. For a long time, we have been warned about the nasty effects of the sun: sunburn, skin cancer and melanoma. The “Slip, Slop, Slap” campaign has focused on avoiding the sun: unfortunately, the pendulum has swung too far the other way. People are now becoming vitamin D deficient, which is leading to other health problems including hypertension, heart attacks, bone problems, cancer, and immune suppression.

You would think that Australia would not have a problem with vitamin D deficiency: but no, there are problems. People are afraid to go out and if they do, they cover up. People work in factories and offices and are rarely exposed to the sun. There is a large group of Australians, especially in the state of Tasmania, who are vitamin D deficient. Tasmania is the most southern state of Australia.

Other than the sun, there are limited food sources of vitamin D. The best source is liver. Animals make vitamin D and store it in the liver. Our ancestors ate all parts of the hunted animals, including the organs. Today, we eat the meat but rarely eat the organs.

Magnesium (Mg) is another important mineral that has close ties with vitamin D and insulin and therefore to high BP.

Mg is a mineral involved in many functions; it is a cofactor in over 300 enzyme reactions, including improving insulin sensitivity, insulin secretion and vascular tone (Gröber, Schmidt, & Kisters, 2015).

A deficiency of Mg produces muscle cramps and spasms. Arteries have muscles in their walls, and it is clear that if the arterial muscles spasm up, then the diameter of the artery narrows, which means the heart must beat harder and BP rises to push blood through the narrowed artery.

Mg is an intracellular mineral and insulin is needed to push Mg into the cells. If there is hyperinsulinaemia, you may think that would push more Mg into the cells. However, that is not the case. This is because where there is hyperinsulinaemia, there is generally an associated IR. IR means that the cells are non-responsive to insulin and Mg does not enter the cells, rather, it stays in the blood, and is eliminated through the urine, which leads to Mg deficiency.

This is the connection between hyperinsulinaemia, IR and Mg deficiency.

Another popular type of anti-hypertensive drug is the calcium channel blockers. Houston (2011) states that Mg is a “natural” calcium channel blocker.

Compounding the Mg deficiency dilemma is food production, preparation, and the diet itself.

Soils are Mg deficient; food refining and manufacture will deplete Mg and the modern generation eats very few greens anyway. The diet, generally, is high in refined carbohydrates, which is low in Mg, which, in turn stimulates insulin Eventually IR develops and what little Mg is obtained in the diet will be lost through the urine. Then a vicious cycle begins: Mg deficiency induces more IR, and the cycle continues.

Many living today on a western diet are Mg deficient.

Mg deficiency leads to muscle spasm and increased BP.

Mg deficiency also leads to cardiac arrhythmia

which can lead to more heart disease.

Mg absorption occurs in the upper part of the small intestine and efficiency depends on intake. When there is plenty of Mg in the diet, absorption efficiency can be as low as 25% but absorption can increase to 70% if there is a low Mg intake. Vitamin D enhances Mg absorption; therefore, in this western society that has a low Mg intake and is vitamin D deficient and is largely insulin resistant, it is no wonder that there is Mg deficiency.

Mg levels need to be improved, either by:

- improving the diet, adding much more green leafy vegetables and salads, (note that chlorophyll is a chelate of Mg, just like haemoglobin is a chelate of Fe) so anything green: containing chlorophyll, will contain Mg, or
- taking a Mg supplement, either orally or topically, or
- soaking in Epsom salt baths. (Epsom salts is Mg sulphate and Mg can be absorbed through the skin.)

Epidemiological studies have confirmed that a daily high Mg intake is predictive of a lower incidence of type 2 diabetes and hypertension (Paolisso & Barbagallo, 1997).

Schutten, Joosten, de Borst, and Bakker (2018)

wrote *"Low dietary magnesium intake has been associated with an increased risk of developing hypertension in prospective cohort studies. Moreover, clinical trials suggest that magnesium supplementation has blood pressure-lowering effects."*

Antioxidants are protective. Much of the damage done to the arteries is by ***oxidative stress***, so a dietary intake of antioxidants can be helpful and protective.

Oxidative stress: a condition of increased oxidant production characterised by the release of free radicals and resulting in cellular damage.

Free radicals: Short lived, highly reactive molecules that have one or more unpaired electrons that cause cellular damage.

Karatzi et al. (2007) showed that the endothelial dysfunction following the smoking of one cigarette was counterbalanced by the consumption of either red wine or de-alcoholised red wine in healthy smokers. This, of course, does not mean that you drink excess red wine if you smoke! What it does show is that antioxidants counter the acute effects of smoke on the endothelium. A diet high in antioxidants, fresh vegetables - the more colourful, the better, green tea, even dark chocolate and red wine can protect against some of these oxidative stresses on our arteries.

Again, it boils down to what we eat.

As oxidative stress is a major cause of endothelial dysfunction, it makes sense that antioxidants may have a useful role in preventing arterial damage. The idea seems logical, but does it work in reality?

We can divide the answer into two parts: primary prevention and secondary prevention.

Primary vs secondary prevention

Primary prevention is preventing the disease from developing in the first place. Secondary prevention is where heart disease already exists, and the aim is to reduce the extent and/or effects. Both use similar regimes, though primary prevention should start as early as possible to prevent heart disease and hypertension developing. This is especially pertinent if there is a strong family history of heart disease, hypertension, or any of the other manifestations of MetS.

Primary prevention relies on lifestyle changes, including weight loss, exercise, reduction of alcohol consumption, stop smoking, as well as a diet higher in fruits and vegetables, nuts and low in sugar and refined carbohydrates.

Conventionally, pharmaceuticals are used.

"Recent randomized controlled trials have demonstrated that these lifestyle changes can be sustained over long periods of time (more than 3 years) and can have blood pressure-lowering effects as large as those seen in drug studies" (Krousel-Wood, Muntner, He, & Whelton, 2004).

Secondary prevention should also follow the same recommendations. Various minerals, vitamins and herbs can also be used. These minerals and vitamins can be from food; green leafy vegetables for Mg, fresh fruit and vegetables for vitamin C, Brazil nuts for selenium (Se), garlic, fish for fish oil (omega 3 fatty acids), etc. Additionally, the use of supplements can be considered such as vitamin C, vitamin E, coenzyme Q10, and l-arginine.

The use of various supplements has been studied.

Magnesium (Mg)

"A major role for magnesium is in the regulation of blood pressure. While data are not entirely consistent, it does appear that an inverse relationship between magnesium intake and blood pressure is strongest for magnesium obtained from food rather than that obtained via supplements." (Champagne, 2000).

"...magnesium supplementation significantly lowers BP in individuals with insulin resistance, prediabetes, or other noncommunicable chronic diseases." (Dibaba et al., 2017).

Calcium (Ca)

"An increase in calcium intake slightly reduces both systolic and diastolic blood pressure in normotensive people, particularly in young people, suggesting a role in the prevention of hypertension." (Cormick, Ciapponi, Cafferata, Cormick, & Belizán, 2022). In this review, people with normal BP were put into 2 groups: Ca supplementation, or Ca food fortification and placebo or control group. The end point was the development of hypertension.

Vitamin C

"VitC supplementation resulted in a significant reduction of blood pressure in patients with essential hypertension." (Guan, Dai, & Wang, 2020).

Though, Al-Khudairy et al. (2017) states *"In terms of clinical events, only one trial was identified to examine the effects of vitamin C on CVD events for primary prevention. These results are however restricted to middle-aged and older male physicians in the USA."*

Vitamin E

Zhang et al. (2023) showed that vitamin E intake shows a "J" curve. Vitamin E levels were assessed as quintiles, the first and fifth quintile showed higher risks of developing hypertension compared to the second to fourth quintiles. In other words, too low and too high vitamin E levels can be problematic. There is a "Goldilocks' zone".

Foods such as nuts, avocado, salmon, mango, kiwi fruit, broccoli, asparagus, and sunflower seeds are high in vitamin E.

Fish oil

Fish oil, which is high in omega 3 fatty acids, is strongly associated with heart benefits, though Liao et al. (2022) showed inconsistent results. Omega 3 may have benefits with hypertension, coronary artery disease, cardiac arrhythmias, and heart failure.

Fish oils should be part of the treatment, not necessarily a standalone treatment. Eating fresh deep-sea ocean fish is part of a healthy diet. Though be wary about ocean pollution, e.g. Hg.

If fish oil supplements are used, ensure that they are labelled as being Hg free.

A better option is krill oil as it is generally cleaner and more concentrated. Only 1-2 small capsules are needed, not 6-8 large fish oil capsules.

Selenium (Se)

Selenium (Se) is a trace mineral that is required for proper heart function and to prevent oxidative stress (Shimada, Alfulaij, & Seale, 2021).

Ju et al. (2017) wrote *"Selenium supplementation decreased serum CRP and increased the GSH-PX level, suggesting a positive effect on reducing oxidative stress and inflammation in CHD. However, selenium supplementation is not sufficient to reduce mortality and to improve the lipid status."*

A good dietary source of Se is Brazil nuts.

Garlic

Wang, Yang, Qin, and Yang (2015) showed that garlic supplements are superior to placebo in reducing BP.

Ried (2020) showed that garlic can be a standalone, or adjunctive anti-hypertensive treatment, with multiple benefits for cardiovascular health. It is highly tolerable and has a high safety profile.

So, for good health, add garlic to your diet.

Coenzyme Q10

Supplementing coenzyme Q10 (CoQ10) has been shown to have a beneficial effect on BP. A study by Tabrizi et al. (2018) showed benefit with reducing systolic BP but not diastolic pressure. A newer study by

Zhao et al. (2022) showed benefit at 100 – 200 mgs/day of CoQ10. Doses up to 1,200 mg/day have been shown to be safe (Hathcock & Shao, 2006).

L-arginine

L-arginine is an amino acid that is the precursor for nitric oxide (NO) which is one of the main regulators of vascular tone. A supplement of l-arginine has been shown to be effective in reducing BP (Shiraseb et al., 2022).

Hawthorn (*Crataegus spp)*

Hawthorn is a herb that has been used for heart conditions for a very long time. It is particularly useful for congestive heart failure and for management of hypertension (Cloud, Vilcins, & McEwen, 2020).

"...hawthorn extracts exert a wide range of cardiovascular pharmacological properties, including antioxidant activity, positive inotropic effect, anti-inflammatory effect, anticardiac remodeling effect, antiplatelet aggregation effect, vasodilating effect, endothelial protective effect, reduction of smooth muscle cell migration and proliferation, protective effect

against ischemia/reperfusion injury, antiarrhythmic effect, lipid-lowering effect and decrease of arterial blood pressure effect" (Wang, Xiong, & Feng, 2013).

Diet

Epidemiological studies have shown that diet, especially the Mediterranean diet, can prevent heart disease. Diet is important. A study, discussed by Simopoulos, and Robinson, (1998), looked at 12,000 men from Greece, Italy, the Netherlands, Finland, Yugoslavia, Japan, and the USA, found that the healthiest were living on the island of Crete. On further study, the traditional Cretan diet, which has been unchanged for thousands of years, was found to be high in antioxidants found in fresh fruit and vegetables, and fats, especially omega 3 fatty acids. The Cretan diet had an omega 3 to omega 6 ratio of 1 to 4. The cancer rate in these men was half that of the USA and the coronary death rate was one twentieth of the USA. Even though the content of fat in the diet was 40% they were obviously doing the right thing. They must be eating the right foods and that includes the "right" fats.

de Lorgoril et al. (1998) tested the Mediterranean diet in men with newly diagnosed cancer and who also had cardiovascular disease and compared it to the "prudent" diet recommended by the American Heart Association (AHA). The group on the Mediterranean diet had a much better survival rate.

The Lyon Diet Heart Study tested a Mediterranean diet on male survivors after the first heart attack. The group was divided into two groups: the Mediterranean diet and a control group. The resultant data showed the dietary modifications were protective (de Lorgoril et al. 1997).

In the final report, after a four year follow up, de Lorgoril et al. (1999) concluded *that "The protective effect of the Mediterranean dietary pattern was maintained up to 4 years after the first infarction, confirming previous intermediate analyses."*

Singh et al. (2017) defined the Mediterranean diet as being *"distinguished by a beneficial fatty acid profile that is rich in both monounsaturated and polyunsaturated fatty acids, high levels of polyphenols and other antioxidants, high intake of fiber and other low glycemic carbohydrates, and relatively greater vegetable than animal protein intake. Specifically, olive oil, assorted fruits, vegetables, cereals, legumes, and nuts; moderate consumption of fish, poultry, and red wine; and a lower intake of dairy products, red meat, processed meat and sweets…*"

Sudden cardiac death (SCD) is a major issue in western society. A large proportion of heart deaths occur in non-hospital situations; the first sign that there is a problem is when the person collapses and drops dead. The major cause of this SCD is due to ventricular arrhythmia, notably ventricular fibrillation (85% of the time). Fish oil, in the form of regular fish consumption, or the supplementation of fish oil has been shown to reduce SCD dramatically.

The GISSI trial (**G**ruppo **I**taliano per lo **S**tudio della **S**opravvivenza nell'**I**nfarcto miocardio) showed significant results: 1 gram of omega 3 fatty acid was beneficial for prevention of death and for combined death, non-fatal myocardial infarction, and stroke. All the benefit was attributable to the decrease in risk for overall (-20%), cardiovascular (-30%) and sudden death (-45%). They concluded that even though fish oil does not have any cholesterol lowering ability, it is a relevant pharmacological treatment for secondary prevention after myocardial infarction (Marchioli et al., 2005).

Note: fish oil also has anti-inflammatory activity.

What I found amusing is that the researchers refer to fish oil as a "drug" as well as referring to it as a "pharmacological treatment."

Fish oil is a natural nutrient, not a drug.

Another arrhythmia that is common, especially among the elderly is atrial fibrillation (AF). Fish oil, in the form of eating fish and presumably, fish oil supplementation, has been shown to reduce the incidence of AF. What is interesting was that the researchers found benefit with consumption of tuna or other broiled or baked fish but not with fried fish or fish sandwiches (Mozaffarian et al., 2004).

However, a newer study (Zhang et al 2022) indicated that fish oil may increase the risk of AF. However, the risk was greater in those taking more than 1 gram per day. (Gencer, Djousse, Al-Ramady, Cook, Manson, & Albert, 2021).

Extramiana and Leenhardt, (2022) queried this result. This could be a case of association, rather than causation. Fish oil is well known to be of benefit on cardiovascular morbidity and mortality.

Another nutrient that can be used to treat arrhythmia is Mg. I recently saw a patient who develops recurrent attacks of AF. He told me that the last time he went to hospital with AF, they immediately put up a Mg infusion.

A similar study showed that eating fish, again tuna or other broiled or baked fish but not fried fish or fish sandwiches, lowered the incidence of congestive cardiac failure (CCF) (Mozaffarian, Bryson, Lemaitre, Burke, & Siscovick, 2005).

Omega 3 fatty acids, in the form of eating fish or as a fish oil supplement, are essential for heart health. Our ancestors evolved on a diet with an omega 3 to omega 6 ratio, in the order of 1:1 to 1:4. However the modern western diet has an omega 3 to omega 6 ratio approximately 1:40. There is too much omega 6 (and/or not enough omega 3) because of the popularity of grains and cereals and the plant polyunsaturated oils. These "foods" are promoted because they are "cholesterol free" and are thought to be protective. They do the opposite. They make the situation worse. What humans need to do is to reduce the omega 6 and to increase omega 3 intake.

An animal living and eating its natural diet will produce omega 3 in its body. If a hunter then eats that animal, they will get the benefit of the omega 3. So, our hunter-gatherer ancestors hunted free range animals and obtained the benefit. However, today, farmed animals do not eat their normal diet. They are grain fed, they are fed pellets, more than likely based on grain, therefore, these farmed animals have a higher omega 6 content.

A free-range chicken eats what chickens normally eat; they scratch around and eat grubs and whatever. These free-range chickens have a better omega 3 to 6 ratio. A free-range chicken laid egg also has a higher omega 3 content as compared to the battery hen which is pellet fed.

So, as a part of a cardio-protective diet, eat free range eggs and meat, organic vegetables and salads and fruits. This will maximise your omega 3 intake and reduce the added chemicals, pesticides, and herbicides found in commercial produce as already discussed. This will also reduce insulin stimulation and help improve IR.

It can be particularly useful and positive to suggest to patients who are suffering from any form of heart disease to increase their fish oil consumption. Whether they choose to do this through supplementation, or by increasing dietary fish intake, is a matter of preference.

> *"Just as food causes chronic disease, it can be the most powerful cure."*
> **Hippocrates (c460 - c370 BCE)**

A cardio-protective lifestyle, which includes a diet high in antioxidants and fish oil, with sensible supplementation, as well as more exercise, more sunshine (vitamin D) and more sleep, can bring positive results.

Treating BP with conventional medications initially is advisable because high BP can cause increased morbidity and mortality. However, if the underlying metabolism, hyperinsulinaemia and IR are treated early, before hypertension develops, then this would have a preventative effect such that medication probably may not be necessary.

When elevated BP is detected, treatment to reduce BP is needed. However, if, at the same time, the above changes to diet and lifestyle, as well as introduction of specific nutrients, herbs, and supplements are started, then as BP improves, the pharmaceutical medication can be slowly reduced with a view of completely stopping if and when the BP has normalised. However, it is important to continue to monitor the BP and immediately intervene should the BP rise again.

CANCER

"In my practice as surgeon, I am impressed by the alarming increase of cancer cases brought to my notice; an increase, which in the light of the general hygienic and sanitary improvements of our time, can point to no other cause than the indulgence in certain foodstuffs detrimental to normal life of the body."

Charles Horace Mayo (1865 – 1939)

Cancer is generally not recognized as being included in the "Deadly Quartet", yet it should be, and the name changed to the "Deadly Quintet".

Cancer is related to hyperinsulinaemia and is therefore a **disease of civilization**.

Cancer has become the number one killer in Australia; and this probably would also be similar in the western world generally.

(https://www.cancer.org.au/cancer-information/what-is-cancer/facts-and-figures - Accessed 30 August 2023)

In 1900, cancer was number eight on the list of causes of mortality.

The rates of cancer have greatly increased over the last 100 years, as well as the age of onset.

Zhao et al. (2023) showed that early onset cancer morbidity continues to increase (i.e., cancer developing at a younger age). The researchers concluded that *"Encouraging a healthy lifestyle could reduce early-onset cancer disease burden."*

Cancer was known from ancient times, so it is not a new disease, but what is new, is the increasing incidence, and at a younger age.

Cancer has been found among fossilized bones, ancient Egyptian mummies, and was described in ancient manuscripts. The oldest description of cancer was from Ancient Egypt, approximately 1600 BCE.

Hippocrates (c460 - c370 BCE) introduced the term *carcinos* and *carcinoma.*

The incidence of cancer in the past is not known for sure but it was exceptionally low, much lower than it is now. Accurate statistics were not started till the 1930s. In 1900, approximately 3% of deaths were caused by cancer; today the incidence of death due to cancer is approximately 20% (one in five deaths).

Why?

The causes of cancer are complex and multi-factorial, and much is not known, so it would be presumptuous of me to indicate that I have all the answers. What I will discuss is the role of civilization in the development of cancer. Cancer is a **disease of civilization**. It is related to diet, lifestyle, drugs, toxic heavy metals, pollution, and chemicals on our contaminated planet.

Definition

Cancer is a disease of the cells, which are the body's basic building blocks. Cancer occurs when abnormal cells grow in an uncontrolled way. These abnormal cells can damage or invade the surrounding tissues, or spread to other parts of the body, causing further damage.

(https://www.canceraustralia.gov.au/impacted-by-cancer/what-cancer. - Accessed 30 August 2023)

This unregulated growth is caused by a series of acquired or inherited mutations to DNA within cells.

This results in damaged genetic information that defines the cell functions and removal of normal control of cell division.

Growth of cell numbers is a normal phenomenon. We all start as a single cell fertilized ovum and we grow into a baby and then into an adult, so growth of cell numbers is a necessary part of living and growing.

There is also a mechanism for cells to die called *apoptosis*. This is a part of the *yin-yang* cycle of life. Normal cell numbers grow to a predetermined point and then stop. Cells wear out, get damaged and die; these are replaced. This is a normal part of life.

Cancer is where the growth is uncontrolled, and/or the death of cells is reduced. More than likely a bit of both happens.

What causes cells to become abnormal? This is the topic of ongoing and continuing research and study. Some factors have been identified and include genetics, diet, viral infection, radiation, chemicals, pollutants, and drugs. The exact biochemical mechanisms are not clear.

In line with the theme of this book so far, I will start by looking at diet.

Primitive cultures did develop cancer, but it was exceedingly rare. These people were not immune to cancer, and this is shown by the increase in cancer rates with the introduction of a western diet.

When Dr Albert Schweitzer first went to Gabon in 1913, there were no known cases of cancer. However, he noted sadly that: *"In the course of the years we have seen cases of cancer in growing numbers in our region. My observations incline me to attribute this to the fact that the natives were living more and more after the manner of the whites . . ."*

Diet does have a role to play in the development of cancer.

What specifically is the harmful factor in the diet?

We can start off with the main theme of this book: hyperinsulinaemia, which is caused by a refined carbohydrate diet. There are other factors, such as alteration of the insulin-like growth factor system, inflammation, abnormalities of the sex hormone metabolism, air pollution, desynchronisation of the circadian rhythm and endocrine disruptors, which can be related to MetS (Bellastella, Scappaticcio, Esposito, Giugliano, & Maiorino, 2018).

I have already stated that the development of cancer is multifactorial, which includes the environment; but that environment must interact with a genetic susceptibility.

Both are important.

If the genetic susceptibility is strong, then there needs to be only a little environmental effect. If there is little or no genetic susceptibility, cancer can still develop where there is a powerful environmental stimulus.

Cancer cells are produced regularly; however, a strong immune system can detect these cells and destroy them before they can proliferate. This is referred to as the immune surveillance theory and relies on a strong immune system. Anything that can suppress the immune system can possibly predispose to the development of cancer. The immune system needs to be protected.

Immune suppression can develop as a consequence of chronic inflammation. Since MetS is associated with chronic inflammation, it can be a cause of cancer (Wu, Dong, Duan, Zhu & Deng, 2017).

Having a genetic susceptibility does not necessarily mean that cancer will develop. This is like being sent an email with an attached virus. The virus will not infect your computer unless you open the attachment. That virus could sit in your inbox for a long time, un-opened and no harm is done. The virus will only be unleashed if something happens, e.g. you open the attachment.

With genetic susceptibility, you may have the programme but unless you activate it, cancer does not necessarily develop. Diet, nutritional status, lifestyle, and chemicals are among some of the factors that can activate that cancer programme. Conversely, diet and lifestyle can protect from developing cancer.

The development of certain cancers is related to elevated levels of plasma insulin-like growth factor-1 (IGF-1) and reduced levels of insulin-like growth factor binding protein-3 (IGFBP-3).

IGF-3 has a direct mitogenic effect on neoplastic cells and an anti-apoptotic effect (apoptosis is the programmed cell death).

IGFBP-3 has an apoptotic action on prostate cells, breast cells and other cell types.

Where is the connection with hyperinsulinaemia?

Insulin, itself, has a stimulating effect on cell growth.

Hyperinsulinaemia, induced by a high glycaemic, refined carbohydrate diet causes increases in IGF-1 and reduction in IGFBP-3.

This reduction of IGFBP-3 is probably related to reduced synthesis caused by the effect hyperinsulinaemia and IR have on liver function.

IGFBP-3 also influences retinoid receptor activity. Retinoids are basically vitamin A and the connection between deficiency of vitamin A and the development of cancer, especially prostate and cervical cancer, is well known. Therefore, if there is any interference with retinoid receptor activity, this would stimulate the activity of IGF-1 and enhance unregulated tissue growth.

As we have seen, a high sugar, high refined carbohydrate diet can lead to hyperinsulinaemia.

Hyperinsulinaemia and sugar

We can lump sugar and hyperinsulinaemia into the same category. Many studies have been done looking at sugar in the diet, while some other studies have looked at hyperinsulinaemia.

Is cancer development due to the sugar or to the resultant hyperinsulinaemia? Do we really need to differentiate between the two? One can lead to the other.

Studies have looked at hyperinsulinaemia and were found to have a relationship to cancer development. There is a link between type 2 diabetes and cancer of the colon, liver, pancreas, breast, and endometrium. This appears to be due to the long period of hyperinsulinaemia that precedes type 2 diabetes.

"Measures to decrease insulin levels, including lifestyle improvement and supplementation with agents known to decrease insulin resistance may therefore offer a general approach to prevention of cancer in a wide variety of organ sites of major clinical importance" (Moore, Park, & Tsuda, 1998).

The British Women's Heart and Health Study concluded that hyperinsulinaemia is positively associated with breast cancer amongst the older women participants in this study (Lawlor, Smith, & Ebrahim, 2004). This is confirmed in a newer study (Dong, Wang, Shen, & Chen, 2021).

Studies have also examined the link between hyperinsulinaemia and cancers in men.

In 2005, Hammarsten and Högstedt wrote that *"... hyperinsulinaemia and five other previously established components of metabolic syndrome are shown to be prospective risk factors for deaths that can be ascribed to prostate cancer. These findings confirm previous study, which indicate that prostate cancer is a component of metabolic syndrome. Moreover, these data indicate that hyperinsulinaemia and other metabolic disorders precede deaths caused by prostate cancer.*

Thus, our data support the hypothesis that hyperinsulinaemia is a promoter of clinical prostate cancer. Furthermore, our data suggest that the insulin level could be used as a marker of prostate cancer prognosis and tumour aggressiveness, regardless of the patient's prostate cancer stage, cancer grade and PSA level."

So, this means that if you are obese, diabetic, hypertensive, or have any of the other hallmarks of MetS, then you are more likely to develop cancer.

Certainly, obese men have a higher incidence of prostate cancer, as well as a higher chance of a more aggressive cancer than non-obese men (Freedland et al., 2005).

Is it the hyperinsulinaemia? Or is it the sugar? Is it the obesity? Is it the reduced immune system function? Does it really matter when they are all inter-related? One does lead to the other.

We do know that insulin is an anabolic hormone that encourages cellular growth. Since cancer is a disease of excess cellular growth, the last thing you want is to encourage more growth.

What about sugar?

La Vecchia, Franceschi, Dolara, Bidoli, and

Barbone (1993) performed a simple experiment. They looked at patients with colon cancer and stratified them according to the number of teaspoons of sugar they put in their coffee. Compared to those who used no sugar, they found higher incidences of cancer in those who used three spoonful's of sugar, which was higher than those who used two spoons, and which was higher than those who used one spoonful.

If you are thinking it is not the sugar but the coffee, Tavani et al. (1997) showed that drinking coffee had a protective effect against colon cancer.

Llaha et al. (2021) showed a positive association between sugar-sweetened beverages and colorectal and pancreatic cancer, fruit juices and breast, colorectal and pancreatic cancer and artificial-sweetened beverages and pancreatic cancer risk.

Laguna et al. (2021) concluded *"Simple sugar intake in drinks and fruit juice was associated with an increased risk of overall cancer incidence and mortality and all-cause mortality. This suggests that sugary beverages are a modifiable risk factor for cancer and all-cause mortality."*

Debras et al. (2020) showed that total and added sugar is related to cancer, especially breast cancer, and can be a modifying factor in cancer prevention.

Franceschi et al. (1997) looked at different food groups and the risk of colorectal cancer. They found increasing trends with bread and cereal dishes, potatoes, cakes and desserts and refined sugars. There was no increase nor a decrease with eggs and meat.

This finding, i.e. sugars and carbohydrates in diet related to colon cancer, was confirmed by Franceschi, Favero, Parpinel, Giacosa, and La Vecchia (1998). This same study also confirmed that vegetables provide cancer protection.

One of the worst cancers is pancreatic cancer. The pancreas lies deep in the abdomen, so by the time it presents and is diagnosed, it can be quite advanced. People succumb very quickly after diagnosis. Pancreatic cancer has been shown to be related to hyperinsulinaemia (Zhang et al., 2023).

Obesity and cancer

Obesity is a symptom of MetS. It is the underlying metabolism that causes the cancer and not obesity *per se*.

However, Avgerinos, Spyrou, Mantzoros, and Dalamaga (2019) showed that excess body weight is associated with increased risk of endometrial, oesophageal, renal, and pancreatic adenocarcinomas, gastric cardia, meningioma, multiple myeloma, colorectal, postmenopausal breast, ovarian, gallbladder and thyroid cancers. The mechanism behind this is related to IR, abnormalities of the IGF-system and signalling, sex hormone biosynthesis and pathway, subclinical chronic inflammation, and oxidative stress, as well as alterations in adipokine pathophysiology.

Pati, Irfan, Jameel, Ahmed, and Shahid (2023) showed that 4-8% of cancers are attributed to obesity, especially post-menopausal breast, colorectal, endometrial, kidney, oesophageal, pancreatic liver, and gallbladder cancer. Obesity results in 17% increased risk of cancer-specific mortality. Weight reduction can be an important intervention in cancer care. Though care must be taken because if a cancer patient is losing weight, it may not be a good sign.

Antioxidants

In broad terms, cancer is caused by free radical damage. From this we can extrapolate that taking antioxidants in our diet will be cancer protective. Antioxidants are substances in food that protect tissues from unstable molecules: free radicals. Antioxidants interact with free radicals and stabilize and/or neutralize them. Examples of these substances are beta-carotene, lycopene, and vitamins A, C, and E.

The trace mineral, Se, is also a very important antioxidant and anti-cancer factor. Cancer rates have been correlated with the amount of Se in the soil. The Zlatibor district in Serbia has lower mortality rates of malignant disease and cardiovascular disease compared with other districts in Serbia. Analysis of the water, soil, bedrock, and plants has shown a higher Se content than other areas and this could influence the lower mortality rates (Maksimović, Rsumović, Jović, Kosanović, & Jovanović, 1998).

A similar finding was noted in Texas: the areas of lower Se had higher cancer mortality rates than the higher Se areas (Cech, Holguin, Sokolow, & Smith, 1984). Note that the plant and vegetable content of Se is dependent on the soil content of Se.

We have already seen that a high vegetable diet seems to protect us from developing cancer. Vegetables such as the brassica (broccoli, cauliflower, Brussels sprouts, bok choy, wombok, etc), tomatoes, onions, and garlic, have all been shown to be cancer protective, largely due to the antioxidants and phytochemicals contained within. What is important to note is that vegetables are a whole food, containing many different substances.

Epidemiological studies discussed in this book show that whole foods are protective but what about the individual antioxidants? As we shall see, individual nutrients have not been shown to be as protective. Vitamin C is possibly one exception.

Beta Carotene in food has been shown to be cancer protective, but beta carotene supplements have shown an increase in cancer development (WHO, 2003).

What about mixtures of antioxidants? A study in China (Blot et al., 1993) showed great promise. The people of Linxian Province in China have a very high rate of oesophageal and stomach cancer. Researchers supplemented groups of inhabitants with various combinations of nutrients and found that the combination of beta-carotene, vitamin E and Se reduced the rates of cancer significantly.

Selenium (Se)

Cai et al. (2016) demonstrated that Se supplementation decreased risk of breast cancer, lung cancer, oesophageal cancer, gastric cancer, and prostate cancer, although there was no reduction in the development of skin cancer, colorectal cancer, and bladder cancer. There was, however, a significant reduction in total cancer mortality.

Previous studies of antioxidants only looked at one antioxidant at a time. I have said before that food, like herbs, is a mixture of substances, each combining with their checks and balances, and they work as a whole. Isolating one "active ingredient" may not show benefit.

Lycopene

Lycopene is a carotenoid that gives various fruits and vegetables their red colouring, such as tomato, watermelon, red capsicum, and red cabbage. Although lycopene is a carotenoid, it cannot be converted to vitamin A.

Lycopene as part of tomato consumption has been shown to be protective against prostate cancer (Fraser, Jacobsen, Knutsen, Mashchak, & Lloren, 2020) and against cervical cancer (Ono et al., 2020). However, it is far better eating a whole cooked tomato, preferably organically grown, than taking a lycopene supplement.

Lycopene does not just protect against cancer, but against vascular disease as well. Mazidi, Katsiki, George, and Banach (2020) showed that consuming lycopene as part of eating tomatoes has an overall total, and cardiovascular and cerebrovascular mortality reduction.

Speaking of prostate cancer and diet, Orlich et al. (2020) showed that men who drink more milk tend to have a higher incidence of prostate cancer.

Optimising the diet is still the preferred option. However, the quality of commercially grown food is not good as it is full of chemicals and insecticides and grown in mineral depleted soils. Therefore, to make up for what is missing in commercially grown food, supplements may be a good idea. Consider using organically grown products and free-range meats.

When supplementing, use a mixture of nutrients, as there is no single "silver bullet".

As far as food goes, the most colourful foods are the ones with the most antioxidants. Colour equals antioxidants. Colourful vegetables such as tomatoes, colourful fruit, and berries such as blueberries, and others that are high in colour, such as green tea, and red wine. All colourful and all high in antioxidants.

Vitamin A/carotenoids

Carotenes, especially the well-known beta carotene, are the yellow colouring found in carrots, squash, and a host of other vegetables. Broccoli has a very high level of beta carotene and would be yellow if it wasn't for the (green) chlorophyll.

The importance of this nutrient is that it is converted to vitamin A. About 30 of the 600 identified carotenoids can be converted to vitamin A, mainly in the intestinal wall and the liver. Beta carotene has the highest pro-vitamin A activity. Beta carotene is an antioxidant in its own right.

Beta carotene conversion to vitamin A needs other nutrients such as vitamin C, Zn, and thyroid hormone. The beta carotene to vitamin A conversion is approximately 12 to 1, meaning that 12 mg of beta carotene is converted to 1 mg of vitamin A. The conversion is regulated so that excess doses of beta carotene will not cause toxic levels of vitamin A. Excess beta carotene may turn the person's skin yellow/orange (carotenoderma) but is not dangerous.

There are many conditions that interfere with the conversion of carotenoids in plant foods to vitamin A, including,

- Being an infant or child
- Diabetes
- Low Thyroid Function
- Low Fat Intake

- Intestinal Roundworms
- Diarrhoea
- Pancreatic Disease
- Celiac Disease
- Sprue

Preformed vitamin A is found in liver, cheese, eggs, oily fish, milk, and yoghurt. Preformed vitamin A in high doses can be toxic and teratogenic. Acute toxicity occurs with doses in the order of 25,000 IU per kilogram: e.g., a 100 kg person will need to ingest 2,500,000 IU (that is a huge dose!)

A dose of 250,000 IU Vitamin A given infrequently is safe. The World Health Organization (WHO) gives doses of 200,000 IU in Africa (100,000 IU for children 9-11 months).

Chronic toxicity occurs after ingesting 25,000 IU daily for prolonged periods of time (months to years).

Vitamin A has many functions. It is,

- essential for good vision,
- necessary for reproductive system,
- important in protecting mucous membranes and helping in immune function. Therefore, this vitamin is needed

for normal cellular growth and differentiation, especially for epithelial cells,
- necessary for skin and for any cells that line the opening of the body, nose, mouth, stomach, gut, vagina, urinary tract, and cervix,
- necessary for bone formation, and
- prevents dry skin.

Beta carotene and vitamin A are antioxidants and therefore protects against free radical damage, which is possibly the underlying basis of cancer formation.

There is good evidence that the antioxidant activity of vitamin A will *prevent* cancer development but there is less evidence that vitamin A will *treat* the cancer once it has developed. Reichman et al. (1990) found a lower level of vitamin A in the blood in prostate cancer cases than in those who did not develop cancer.

In another study, this time looking at cervical cancer, Zhang, Dai, Zhang, and Wang (2012) found that dietary vitamin A and serum vitamin A levels were inversely related to risk of cervical cancer.

Although this is probably related more to overall vegetable intake rather than beta carotene itself. Simply supplementing beta carotene has shown poor results, while supplementing beta carotene with other nutrients showed much better results. This highlights the principle of cancer protection coming from a mixture of nutrient/antioxidants, rather than just the one nutrient.

There is no “silver bullet”. As shown above in the study in Linxian Province, China, the combination of beta carotene, vitamin E and Se had significant benefits.

Another nutrient that is related to the cervix is folate. Li et al. (2020) showed that women with a folate deficiency have an increased risk of CIN (cervical intraepithelial neoplasia) and cervical cancer. Though just supplementing folate did not seem to have any anti-cancer benefits. It seems that folate can prevent cervical cancer but not treat it.

Here again, low folate levels would be related more to an overall reduction in fresh fruit and vegetables in the diet, rather than a deficiency of folate *per se.* What we should do is to increase the dietary fruit and vegetables rather than just give a folate supplement. If supplements are used then a mixture is needed, not just an individual nutrient.

However, we are assuming that the person can use dietary folate normally. The methyl tetrahydrofolate reductase (MTHFR) gene is needed for proper folate activation. Some people inherit a variation of this gene. A single nucleotide polymorphism (SNP "snip") of the MTHFR gene may predispose to cervical cancer because of its abnormal folate metabolism. Gong, Shen, Shan, and He (2018) showed that a C667T SNP of the MTHFR gene did not predispose to cervical cancer, however the A1298C SNP did predispose to cervical cancer and CIN. Genetic testing may be useful.

Vitamin C

Despite what I have said above about not relying on individual nutrients, vitamin C on its own has been shown to help protect against cancer, as well as in the treatment of cancer. Intravenous vitamin C has been shown to increase survival in cancer patients compared to historical controls. Casciari et al. (2001) discussed that oral vitamin C did not show benefit because oral vitamin C cannot reach the high serum peak levels achieved by intravenous vitamin C. However, intravenous vitamin C can elevate levels that are cytotoxic to cancer cells. The addition of other antioxidants, glutathione, and alpha lipoic acid, to the vitamin C has been shown to increase the effectiveness of killing cancer cells.

Intravenous vitamin C plus or minus other antioxidants is a valid treatment for cancer.

Vitamin D

I have said it before, and I will say it again: vitamin D is an essential substance for humans: and the main source of vitamin D is the sun.

Vitamin D is not a dietary nutrient as such and is not related to hyperinsulinaemia It is related to our lifestyle and therefore, any disorder caused by a lack of vitamin D, can be considered a **disease of civilization**.

Humans are currently avoiding the sun. We evolved in the sun, not in a hole under the ground. Sunshine is part of our physiology, but our lifestyle has changed. We spend most of our time indoors, away from the sun. We work long hours in the office or the factory and are shielded from the sun. If we do have spare time, we avoid the sun: we have become sun phobic.

The authorities have started a massive anti-sun campaign. The fear of the sun has been instilled in us and we avoid it like the plague. The “Slip, Slop, Slap” campaign has become very successful, in fact, too successful.

Now we have become vitamin D deficient.

The initial premise is that the sun causes skin cancer and melanoma: it is not as simple as that. Possibly, it is the western diet that is very low in antioxidants that allows the free radicals formed in the skin from sun exposure to cause the cancer, not specifically the sunshine alone.

A study by Hercberg et al. (2007) showed that supplementing antioxidants does not protect against skin cancers, and that there is a difference in effect between men and women. Antioxidant supplements do not seem to have any protective benefit; however, diet does seem to have a protective effect. Millen et al. (2004) showed that a diet rich in vitamin D and carotenoids and low in alcohol reduced the risk of melanoma.

Hughes, van der Pols, Marks, and Green (2006) showed a diet rich in green leafy vegetables may prevent the development of subsequent squamous cell carcinomas (SCC) while consumption of unmodified dairy products, such as whole milk, cheese and yoghurt may increase risk of SCC in susceptible people.

How can the negative effects of antioxidant supplementation be explained? Perhaps “too little, too late”? The Hercberg study only lasted for seven years, and the doses given were relatively low.

A diet high in minerals, including Se, antioxidants and carotenoids does have a positive protective effect on the skin as well as against cancer in general.

Bataille et al. (2005) studied the use of sunbeds in

Europe and showed that sunbathing, sunburn or even sunbed exposure was not associated with melanoma risk. The strongest factors that predisposed to melanoma were skin type and numbers of naevi.

Ancestry can also be a factor. People whose ancestors come from higher latitudes (Scotland, Scandinavia) and move to sunny areas, such as Australia, can develop skin problems. Their skins are not equipped to deal with the strong sunny Australian climate.

Contrary to popular belief, Berwick et al. (2005) showed that sun exposure is associated with increased survival after melanoma diagnosis. Many melanoma patients avoid the sun after diagnosis.

Sunshine produces vitamin D, which is a powerful anti-cancer agent: not just for melanoma but for cancer in general.

Grant (2007) stated that *"These results provide nearly direct evidence that solar UVB irradiance reduces the risk of many internal cancers. The likely mechanism is production of Vitamin D."*

So, the crux of the matter is "not too much, not too little." Unfortunately, we have gone from one extreme to the other.

The vitamin D council recommends that you go

out in the summer sun in your bathing suit until your skin just begins to turn pink. This will make, on average 20,000IU of Vitamin D in your skin. That means a few minutes in the summer sun produces 100 times more vitamin D than the government says you need. You cannot become vitamin D toxic from the sun because once you make about 20,000 units, the same ultraviolet light will begin to degrade it. The more you make, the more is destroyed. So, a steady state is reached that prevents the skin from making too much vitamin D.

Lappe, Travers-Gustafson, Davies, Recker, and Heaney (2007) showed that vitamin D (1,100 IU) and Ca supplementation (1400-1500 mgs) can reduce cancer rates by 77%. Although this study was relatively small (1,179 women) and only lasted four years, the results were quite significant.

This may not be a cure for cancer, but prevention is better.

> *"Prevention is better than a cure."*
> **Desiderius Erasmus (1466-1536)**

Environmental chemicals and pollution

We live in a dirty world.

The world is full of chemicals: either as the primary product, or as a by-product of industry. Some chemicals we inadvertently get exposed to simply by living in this polluted world. Other chemicals we purposefully expose ourselves to such as smoking, eating processed foods and by using cosmetics and other personal care products. These chemicals cause havoc to our health. Many of these substances are toxic to the human species; many also act as a hormone blocker/mimicker. These pollutants can cause many varied problems from infertility to cancer.

The clean environment our species evolved in is now full of toxic chemicals and other poisons and our system has not (yet) learned to deal with them. Our liver is working overtime to remove as many toxins as possible.

Cancer caused by chemicals or pollution in our environment is not new. The famous English surgeon, Percivall Potts (1714-1788) was the first to link cancer with a substance in the environment. In 1775 he described a cluster of cases of scrotal cancer amongst chimney sweeps. This was the first report of chemical carcinogenesis.

Since then, many cases of chemical carcinogenesis have been described; perhaps the most well-known is the link between cigarette smoking and lung cancer.

Høyer, Jørgensen, Brock, and Grandjean (2000) showed a link between breast cancer and organochlorine insecticides and herbicides, such as dieldrin, lindane, hexachlorobenzene and dichlorodiphenyltrichloroethane (DDT).

Warner et al. (2002) demonstrated that dioxin is implicated with the development of breast cancer.

Dioxin is the common name for the group of compounds classified as polychlorinated dibenzodioxins (PCDDs). PCDDs, which are members of the family of halogenated organic compounds and have been shown to be bio-accumulative in humans and animals due to their lipophilic properties, and are known to be teratogenic, mutagenic, and carcinogenic (Rathna, Varjani, & Nakkeeran, 2018).

Agent Orange, the chemical defoliant used indiscriminately during the Vietnam war, is a mixture of two chemicals, 2,4, dichlorophenoxyacetic acid (2,4-D) and 2,4,5 trichlorophenoxyacetic acid (2,4,5-T). These two chemicals degraded within days to weeks but there was a toxic contaminant, dioxin, which does not degrade and remains toxic for a very long time. This is now being linked to birth defects (Ngo, Taylor, Roberts, & Nguyen, 2006) and cancer (Chang, Benson, & Fam, 2017) amongst Vietnamese citizens, Vietnam veterans and anyone else who encountered this chemical.

The everyday ritual of applying cosmetics can lead to health issues. The skin is the largest organ in the body. Applying these cosmetic chemicals to the skin for prolonged periods, can result in damage. These compounds are toxic and have xenoestrogenic properties which have hormone receptor mimicking and /or blocking abilities. This is why they can be so dangerous.

Balwierz et al. (2023) identified the potential carcinogens in cosmetics as *"parabens (methylparaben, propylparaben, butylparaben, and ethylparaben), ethoxylated compounds (laureth-4, lautreth-7, or ethylene glycol polymers known as PEG), formaldehyde donors (imidazolidinyl urea, quaternium 15, and DMDM hydantoin), and ethanolamine and their derivatives (triethanolamine and diazolidinyl urea), as well as carbon and silica."*

Other chemicals have endocrine disrupting properties.

"This is due to many substances in cosmetics and sunscreens that have endocrine active properties which affect reproductive health, but which also have other

endpoints, such as cancer" (Nicolopoulou-Stamati, Hens, & Sasco, 2015).

Taylor et al. (2018) looked at the association between personal care product use and breast cancer. The ironic thing is that women recovering from breast cancer treatment are advised to go and have a "makeover" to make them "feel better". This involves applying carcinogenic chemicals to their body. As if they haven't already had enough troubles with cancer.

Pesticide exposure is another possible risk factor for several childhood cancers, particularly acute leukaemia. Mancini et al. (2023) studied children living near areas of vine growing. These vineyards are subject to intense pesticide use. The researchers found a correlation between the development of leukaemia in children and environmental exposure to pesticides.

Another important carcinogenic link is between asbestos and mesothelioma. This link has now been proven conclusively (Gariazzo, Gasparrini, & Marinaccio, 2023).

Also, who can forget the link between hexavalent chromium and cancer that was highlighted in the film *Erin Brockovich*?

More and more connections are being discovered.

We can also look at chemicals in our food. Chemicals included are the insecticides, pesticides, preservatives, colours, flavourings, etc. Many of these compounds are fat soluble and therefore accumulate in fatty tissue. They do not degrade easily and therefore tend to remain in the environment for a very long time.

Any additives or chemicals can be avoided by eating fresh produce, organically grown (which are pesticide, herbicide and chemical free), and not from commercial growers, a packet, or a tin.

Another chemical used in many manufactured foods is aspartame, the artificial sweetener. Landrigan and Straif (2021) showed that aspartame caused cancer in rats. Debras et al. (2022) showed this may also occur in humans.

Heavy Metals (HMs), such as cadmium (Cd), mercury (Hg), lead (Pb), and arsenic (As), have been already mentioned: they are becoming more and more prevalent in this polluted world of ours. HMs come from many sources: industry, mining, and many products found around the home, although many of these sources are now diminishing. There was Pb in the paint and in the solder in the canning industry. Some older paints contained Hg and acted as an anti-fungal agent. Just recently, many products made in China were recalled because of lead-based paint.

Cd is found in cigarette smoke and from the chimneys of incinerators and from coal fired power stations.

There is Hg in dental amalgam fillings, although they are used much less today; however, there is still a large number of people with old amalgam filling. Hg was previously used in vaccines; now largely removed. Aluminium (Al) is found in deodorants, in cookware, and in vaccines.

Many products are eventually dumped, and these toxic heavy metals can leach into groundwater which we will eventually drink.

Seas are polluted and therefore, so are the fish. Eating fish is regarded as being generally a healthy thing to do but can be hazardous due to contamination.

Toxic heavy metal poisoning, especially with Cd, As, beryllium (Be), Hg have been implicated with cancer development (Järup, 2003).

A significant source of Cd is tobacco smoke. This makes tobacco smoking a double whammy.

Cd has an oestrogenic effect and can produce hormone-related cancers and disease in the uterus and the breasts.

Rapisarda et al. (2018) showed that Cd also has an association with the development of prostate cancer.

The development of the chemical industry has produced thousands of different chemicals, in line with the concept of *"better life through chemistry"*. Unfortunately, very little research was done on their long-term effects. Many of these substances are now coming back and biting us on the bum!

The following article says it all so well. This is not only happening in China but probably all over the western, industrialized world.

A report from China *"Pollution and Chemicals blamed for massive cancer rate rise across China"* (Beijing (AFP) May 21, 2007)

"Pollution and the excessive use of chemicals in foodstuffs are sending cancer rates soaring in China, where it is already the number one killer, state press said Monday. Cancer was the most lethal disease in both urban and rural areas last year, the China Daily said, citing a recent health ministry survey."

"The main reason behind the rising number of cancer cases is that pollution of the environment, water and air is getting worse by day," the paper quoted Chen Zhizhou, a cancer expert at the Chinese Academy of

Medical Sciences, as saying.

"Many chemical and industrial enterprises are built along rivers so that they can dump waste into water easily... the contaminated water has directly affected soil, crops and food".

Excessive use of fertilisers and pesticides also pollute underground water, he said, while farmers are using additives on pigs, poultry and vegetables to make them grow faster.

Air pollution is a major cause of lung cancers, as harmful granules enter the lungs and cannot be discharged, the report said.

Large amounts of formaldehyde and related compounds also are widely used in home renovation materials and furniture, further polluting the air in homes.

"A high rate of cancer deaths has become a reality in areas where the environment is heavily polluted," the paper said, citing numerous examples of "cancer villages" in China that have high rates of deaths attributed to the disease."

Drugs

Drugs are chemicals as well. These chemicals are given by mainstream doctors to cure disease. In some cases, the "cure" can be worse than the disease.

> *"The best doctor gives the least medicines."*
> Benjamin Franklin (1706-1790)

Who can forget the diethylstilboestrol (DES) fiasco?

This oestrogenic drug was given to millions of women, all over the world from 1938 to the 1970s to prevent miscarriages, yet in the end, was shown to be useless for that purpose.

Not only did the DES increase the chance of developing breast cancer in the mother taking the DES, but also increased the chance of developing cancer in the daughters exposed to the DES *in utero*. Female foetuses exposed to DES *in utero* had an increased chance of developing clear cell carcinoma of the vagina later in life, while male foetuses had an increased chance of developing genital abnormalities. There is also evidence that the DES daughters are prone to giving birth to male children with increased risk of hypospadias, and daughters with menstrual and obstetric abnormalities; meaning that a third generation is being affected (Gaspari et al., 2023; Titus et al., 2019; Kalfa, Paris, Soyer-Gobillard, Daures, & Sultan, 2011).

The problem will not go away quickly (Klip et al., 2002; Blatt, Van Le, Weiner, & Sailer, 2003; Treffers, Hanselaar, Helmerhorst, Koster, & van Leeuwen, 2001; Titus-Ernstoff et al., 2001).

Hormone replacement therapy (HRT)

The popularity of hormone replacement therapy (HRT) has produced many problems, including cancer.

For years HRT was recommended for women for menopausal problems, as well as heart protection, prevention of Alzheimer's, the reduction of urinary incontinence and, of course, for hot flushes. In the past, many women were put on hormones, not because they had any symptoms, but because they were at the "right age", i.e. menopausal. They were given for prevention of the above conditions. One by one, these effects have been disproved, except for one: the treatment of hot flushes.

The link between HRT and cancer has been known

for a long time, yet largely ignored. For many years, even though the dogma was that oestrogen was protective, studies had shown that women on oestrogen replacement developed heart disease. It was not until the Women's Health Initiative (WHI), a study of 161,809 post-menopausal women with intact uteri, that people really stood up and took notice (Rossouw et al., 2002).

The conclusion of the combined estrogen/progestin arm of the trial was that health risks exceeded benefits from the use of combined oestrogen and progestin over an average of 5.2 years follow up. (Note progestin is a synthetic progesterone analogue.) There was an increase in breast cancer, heart attacks, strokes, and pulmonary emboli. Short-term use is safe for alleviation of hot flushes, but long-term use causes more morbidity and death than what it saves. It goes without saying that hot flushes are uncomfortable, but people do not die of them, while people do die of breast cancer, heart attacks, strokes, etc.

Soon afterwards, the *"Million Women Study"* (Beral et al., 2003) confirmed these findings. HRT is dangerous for women. At present the only use for HRT is for short term treatment of hot flushes (although there are many natural treatments, that are a lot safer, that can deal with these issues). This study not only showed that synthetic oestrogen was dangerous, but that the synthetic oestrogen and progestin combination was even worse.

Breast cancer rates had been increasing but, in 2003, the rates started to drop in the over 50 age group and have continued to drop. So, what happened in 2003? This is the year that the WHI study was released and made front page in nearly every newspaper in the world. Women were frightened, and rightly so. Up to 46% of women stopped taking the HRT.

Katalinic and Rawal (2008) agree that this reduction of breast cancer rates is most likely because hundreds of thousands of women stopped taking HRT. It is not due to any new treatments.

Ravdin et al. (2007) concurred. *"The decrease was evident only in women who were 50 years of age or older and was more evident in cancers that were estrogen-receptor–positive than in those that were estrogen-receptor–negative. The decrease in breast-cancer incidence seems to be temporally related to the first report of the Women's Health Initiative and the ensuing drop in the use of hormone-replacement therapy among postmenopausal women in the United States. The contributions of other causes to the change in incidence seem less likely to have played a major role but have not been excluded."*

I remember speaking with my colleagues and they

were worried and upset because most of their patients had gone off the hormones. My patients thanked me for not starting them on HRT hormones in the first place. I generally used the natural bio-identical hormones (B-HRT). These have been shown to be much safer than HRT (Holtorf, 2009; Moskowitz, 2006).

Fournier, Berrino, and Clavel-Chapelon (2008), in the Etude Epidémiologique auprès de femmes de la Mutuelle Générale de l'Education Nationale (E3N) cohort study showed that breast cancer development can be related more to the use of synthetic progestins, rather than oestrogen. The use of natural progesterone can reduce the risk.

Unopposed oestrogen (that is the use of oestrogen without progesterone) is probably the only cause of uterine cancer and even the addition of a progestins (synthetic progesterone) reduces the risk only minimally (Beresford, Weiss, Voigt, & McKnight, 1997).

Even the use of the contraceptive pill has shown an increase in breast cancer compared to women who had not used them. The risk increased the longer they were used for. The absolute risk however is small (Mørch et al., 2017).

Other drugs commonly used are the proton pump inhibitors (PPIs), which are used to reduce stomach acid.

These were shown to increase the risk of gastric cancer, but not colorectal risk. PPIs should only be used for a short time and in the lowest possible dose. Unfortunately, they are over-used, for extended times and in high doses (Guo et al. 2023).

Statins and cancer have already been discussed.

Another group of drugs that cause cancer are the drugs used to treat cancer. What a paradox!

Anti-cancer drugs are used to kill off cancer cells; they also kill off the immune system. So, if a person with cancer survives the treatment, the drugs and radiation (see next section) that brought about this "cure", they are predisposed to cancer later.

It is ironic that the National Institute for Occupational Safety and Health (NIOSH) released an alert to the nation's 5.5 million health care workers: The powerful drugs used in chemotherapy can themselves cause cancer and pose a risk to nurses, pharmacists and others who handle them.

My comment is ...What about the people receiving these drugs?

> *"The person who takes medicine must recover twice, once from the disease, and once from the medicine."*
> **William Osler (1849 – 1919)**

Radiation

Radiation comes from 3 main sources.

- Natural background radiation from cosmic sources, ground radiation, and the like.
- Non-medical sources, such as atomic bombs. The most obvious examples are the atomic bombs dropped on Hiroshima and Nagasaki. Other examples include atomic bomb testing where military personnel and civilians were exposed to radiation, not just in the USA but in Australia (Maralinga) and the South Pacific. Others include occupational and commercial sources.
- Medical radiation: x-rays, radiotherapy, and nuclear medicine.

Radiation causes cancer. We all know this. Evidence comes from studies of the Japanese atomic bomb survivors, who received massive doses of radiation and developed cancer at a rate of 50% greater than those not exposed.

Of course, massive doses can cause cancer, but few people are exposed to such high doses. What about low doses? According to Professor John Goffman, Professor Emeritus of Molecular and Cell Biology at the University of California (Berkeley), researcher and activist, there is no safe limit. Even the smallest dose can cause harm and the dose of radiation is cumulative (Blackburn, 2021).

There are increased rates of thyroid cancer in women exposed to x-rays either occupationally (dentists/dental assistants) and in those undergoing x-ray examinations in a dose response fashion (Memon, Godward, Williams, Siddique, & Al-Saleh, 2010).

Doody et al. (2000) studied a group of women with scoliosis. As part of their treatment, they had repeated x-ray examinations of their spines. They found that the women, who had on average 24.7 x-ray exposures, had a greater risk of dying of breast cancer than the general population. While examining their spines, their breasts were inadvertently irradiated. There were 77 breast cancer deaths amongst this group, compared with 45.6 deaths expected based on US Mortality Rates. The risk increased significantly with the increased number of x-ray examinations.

Another cancer that is in almost epidemic proportions is leukaemia. This disease was very rare before the 1940s. In 1955, David Hewitt of Oxford University noticed a 50% increase in children dying of leukaemia. Alice Stewart of the University's Department of Preventive Medicine started a survey where she interviewed the mothers of 1,094 children who had died of leukaemia or other cancers and compared them to an equal number of mothers of healthy children. The major difference was the number of x-ray examinations each had experienced. She found that twice as many children born of mothers given a pelvic x-ray died of a malignancy before the age of ten. These x-rays were taken during pregnancy for pelvic measurement, for difficult lies or for multiple births. Most of these problems could have been assessed by a good clinical examination. This practice of x-raying pregnant mothers has now largely stopped and is being replaced by ultrasound examination (Stewart & Kneale, 1970).

Rajaraman et al. (2011) came to a similar conclusion. *"Although the results for lymphoma need to be replicated, all of the findings indicate possible risks of cancer from radiation at doses lower than those associated with commonly used procedures such as computed tomography scans, suggesting the need for cautious use of diagnostic radiation imaging procedures to the abdomen/pelvis of the mother during pregnancy and in children at very young ages."*

There should not be such a thing as a "routine x-ray". X-rays need to be done for a reason and that reason must be a good one. There is no point in doing any x-ray if it does not change your action of treatment. On many occasions, x-rays are done more for a medico-legal reason, not a purely clinical reason.

Mammograms

Unfortunately, there are some "routine" x-rays still done. In the name of prevention and good health, there is a screening test called a mammogram.

Since radiation can cause cancer, how safe are they? How useful are they? Are they a cause, at least in part, of the current epidemic of breast cancer? It is worth pointing out that in the past, mammograms were involved with much higher doses of radiation. Today, with more sensitive films, the doses used are much less but can still be a hazard. Mammography does not make women live longer, and mammography leads to more possible unnecessary mastectomies (Gøtzsche, 2015).

Are cancers that were produced from these large doses of radiation coming now to haunt us?

One of the earliest studies showed that mammograms can produce a 30% reduction in death from breast cancer (Nyström et al., 1993).

This study is still quoted and is the reason why public breast screening programmes were instituted. However, subsequent studies have shown that mammographic screening does not have any benefits at all (Gøtzsche & Olsen, 2000).

In a large study of 34,405 women aged 50-59 years, the women were randomised into 2 groups. One group had mammography and physical examination and the other group only had physical examination. Note: all women were taught breast self-examination (BSE). The results showed that the addition of mammography to physical examination and BSE does not change ultimate cancer mortality (Miller, To, Baines, & Wall, 2000).

Every mammogram involves irradiation of the breast with a dose of x-ray; this could mean a greater chance of developing cancer. If mammograms are done yearly or even second yearly, what effect would this have on the development of breast cancer? It goes without saying that the younger the age routine mammograms are started - the more doses of radiation that the woman receives in her lifetime. Would it cause more cancer than it can detect?

Dr Robert Mendelsohn wrote *"I have been warning women for years that the annual mammographic screening for women without symptoms may produce more cancer than it detects. I haven't been alone. Dr John C. Bailar III, editor-in-chief of the Journal of the National Cancer Institute, made the same point in a 1975 report. His conclusion was supported by numerous studies, which suggested that accumulated x-ray doses in excess of 100 rads over 10 to fifteen years may induce cancer of the breast. Dr Irwin Bross, of the Roswell Park Memorial Institute in Buffalo, New York, also warned a congressional subcommittee in 1978 that the quarter of a million women screened in the NCI-ASC mass screening programme will "in fifteen or twenty years become the victims of the worst iatrogenic (doctor caused) breast cancer epidemic in medical history"* (Mendelsohn, 1982).

In 1995, Wright and Mueller wrote in the Lancet, *"The early trials of screening mammography, reporting 30% relative reduction in mortality from breast cancer in women over 50 years of age, led to strong professional and public demand for screening programmes. There has been little publicity about the subsequent trials showing no significant benefit in any age group, or about the harm and costs associated with screening mammography. For women under 50, there is a reluctant consensus that screening is not beneficial, but there is increasing pressure for publicly funded* *programmes for older women. When analysed in terms of population benefit, the randomised controlled prospective trials showed that the numbers of women screened to achieve one less death per year ranged from 7086 (Health Insurance Plan of New York), to 63,264 (Malmo), to infinity (Canadian National Breast Screening Study). About 5% of screening mammograms are positive or suspicious, and of these 80-93% are false positives that cause much unnecessary anxiety and further procedures including surgery. False reassurance by negative mammography occurs in 10-15% of women with breast cancer that will manifest clinically within a year. Our calculations confirm others that the mean annual cost per life "saved" is around $1-2 million (558,000 pounds). In the allocation of limited resources, public health policy on a proposed mass population intervention must be based on a critical analysis of benefits, harm, and cost. Since the benefit achieved is marginal, the harm caused is substantial, and the costs incurred are enormous, we suggest that public funding for breast cancer screening in any age group is not justifiable."*

The usefulness of mammograms is controversial. They may detect early cancers, but they also detect many non-cancers that lead to surgical and medical intervention, with the associated emotional and financial burden. There is a high incidence of false positives, i.e.

a lesion is found and on biopsy, is not cancerous.

The usefulness of mammograms does depend on age.

The younger age group should not have routine screening mammograms because the dense glandular structure of the young breast makes reading the mammogram difficult. Also, the young breast tissue is extra sensitive to radiation and could lead to long term carcinogenesis. Starting at a younger age exposes the breast to more radiation from the increased numbers of mammograms.

Cancer, especially breast cancer, is now developing at a younger age. There are many factors which will be discussed in this book.

The 40–49-year age group is perhaps one of the controversial groups. This group may benefit from mammograms, though the increasing numbers of ductal carcinoma in situ (DCIS) discovered increases the rate of biopsy and subsequent mastectomy, although this may reduce the need for chemotherapy or radiation. There is a significant false negative rate: 1 in 4 cancers can be missed.

The over 50 age group is also controversial. Eighty percent of all breast cancers occur in women over 50, though perhaps they have been developing for some time. The recommendation is to have yearly or 2 yearly mammograms. In one of the studies quoted above, BSE with physical examination was as good as mammogram.

However, here again, each woman should be looked at individually and not as part of a community-wide blanket screening programme.

Women know their breasts better than anyone else. BSE is important, as women examining their own breasts can detect any changes. Any new lump that is found and doesn't disappear after a period needs further investigation, which would include a mammogram. I have no issues with using mammograms to investigate a breast lump.

Kerlikowske, Salzmann, Phillips, Cauley, and Cummings (1999) showed that in the over 70 age group, there is really no evidence that mammograms offer any major benefits in gains in life expectancy.

Since mammograms came into vogue, the rate of detecting ductal carcinoma in situ (DCIS) has increased dramatically (328%): these are *precancerous* lesions. Figures vary but 30-50% can become cancerous, therefore, conversely, up to 70% may not become cancerous.

What really is not known is which ones become

cancerous. Despite this, they are all treated the same: lumpectomy or mastectomy. However, some opt for a new approach, "watchful waiting". The danger is using frequent mammography to monitor the lesion. Ultrasound or MRI would be a better approach.

Since mammography started, the rate of mastectomy has increased.

At present there is no answer as to which cancers will spread. Defensive action can be taken by losing weight, increasing vitamin D levels, avoiding synthetic hormones, avoiding radiation as much as possible and, of course, keeping your insulin levels low.

There should not be a blanket approach to mammography. The approach should be personalized with each individual woman, considering the age, family history, lifestyle, diet, obesity and if they have taken synthetic hormones.

With all the facts, women can make an informed choice on when and how often they have mammograms. This decision needs to be made in conjunction with their health professional or doctor.

There is a story about a celebrity who was so paranoid about breast cancer, that she had 6-monthly mammograms. After some time, she did develop breast cancer. Could the frequent mammograms have been responsible for this?

The change from mammograms to breast magnetic resonance imaging (MRI) is starting to occur. This is because MRIs do not use radiation. Breast MRIs are recommended for women with a high risk of breast cancer, or a strong family history of breast cancer. The big impediment is the cost. MRIs are not cheap. New abbreviated and ultrafast protocols are being developed. (Heller & Moy, 2019)

Mobile phones

Another source of radiation is the mobile phone: a relatively new phenomenon. There are, therefore, no long-term studies yet, and what studies have been done are contradictory. Mobile phones have become extremely popular: there are over two billion in use all over the world. They are an essential tool, although to some they are a fashion accessory. Mobile phones emit electromagnetic radiation in the microwave range.

There is great controversy about whether they can cause cancer. We see study after study, each contradicting each other.

Yes, or no?

Lahkola et al. (2007) showed that there was some relationship between mobile phone use and the development of glioma (a form of brain cancer). Obviously, this is related to holding the phone next to your head.

An earlier study (Hardell, Mild, & Carlberg, 2003) also showed a relationship between mobile phone and cordless phone use and brain tumours. Note that the cordless phone emits more radiation than a mobile phone.

Breast cancer is uncommon under the age of 50. However, some women are carrying their mobile phones tucked into their bra. These women had their mobile phones in direct contact with skin and breast for up to ten hours every day for years. West et al. (2013) described four case studies where women developed breast cancer, where the scans showed clustering of multiple tumour foci directly under the area of phone contact.

Shih et al. (2020) concluded that *"Excessive smartphone use significantly increased the risk of breast cancer, particularly for participants with smartphone addiction, a close distance between the breasts and smartphone, and the habit of smartphone use before bedtime."*

Hepworth et al. (2006) published a study showing that there was no relationship between mobile phone use and brain cancer. One thing that needs to be pointed out is that this study was partly funded by the manufacturers of mobile phones.

Is there perhaps a conflict of interest?

Mobile phones are big business: this is where politics, finance and health can get mixed up. When these three get together, it is usually health that loses out.

We still do not know for sure. It is best to assume that there may be a risk. Avoid long mobile phone conversations. Use hands free or loudspeaker mode to avoid putting the microwave transmitter next to your head.

The newest study seems to conclude that mobile phone use can cause cancer. Choi, Moskowitz, Myung, Lee, and Hong (2020) concluded that *"This comprehensive meta-analysis of case-control studies found evidence that linked cellular phone use to increased tumor risk."*

Of course, this study has been criticized.

Children really should not use mobile phones but unfortunately, they do, a lot!

Electromagnetic radiation

Electromagnetic radiation is also another issue.

Does electromagnetic radiation from power lines and other electronic equipment cause cancer or any other disease?

This is, of course, again, a very controversial topic.

"There is an association between childhood leukaemia and proximity of home address at birth to high voltage power lines, and the apparent risk extends to a greater distance than would have been expected from previous studies" (Draper, Vincent, Kroll, & Swanson, 2005).

Lowenthal, Tuck, and Bray (2007) came to a similar conclusion *"Although recognizing that this study has limitations, the results raise the possibility that prolonged residence close to high-voltage power lines, especially early in life, may increase the risk of the development of MPD (myeloproliferative disorders) and LPD (lymphoproliferative disorders) later."*

There probably are studies that show no connection.

"When in doubt...don't."
Benjamin Franklin (1706-1790)

The best thing is not to live near high tension power lines, but then, not everyone can choose where they live. High tension power lines usually do not pass through the well-to-do areas but through the low socio-economic areas. This population is already stressed enough and possibly also has poor diets. The electro-magnetic waves are perhaps the final straw.

Stress

Stress causes cancer: everyone knows that! We probably all know someone who succumbed to cancer after a scare, or after the death of a spouse, or some other stressful event. There are many examples of stress and cancer being linked.

From a theoretical point of view, and from laboratory studies, it makes sense. A study in 1983 by Schleifer, Keller, Camerino, Thornton, and Stein, looked at spouses of women with terminal breast cancer. A highly significant suppression of immune function was seen as early as one month after bereavement.

We know that stress influences the hormone system, especially cortisol, which has a profound effect on the immune system.

The stress hormone, adrenaline, has been shown to protect cancer cells from apoptosis (programmed cell death). This action was observed at adrenaline levels found after acute and chronic psychosocial stress. This could be one of the mechanisms by which stress promotes tumour growth and decreases the efficacy of anti-cancer therapies (Sastry et al., 2007).

On the other hand, we know that cancer does not grow overnight. How can we explain a cancer death within six months of the death of a spouse? That cancer must have been there for some time.

We all develop cancer, every day, but our immune system either eliminates it at an early stage before it is allowed to develop or keeps it in check, in a dormant state. Of course, this assumes a very efficient immune system. Any compromise to the immune system will interfere with this cancer monitoring and eliminating function.

In the case where a surviving spouse dies of cancer soon after the death of the partner, the cancer could have been there for years, but the immune system kept it in check. As soon as the stress developed, the immune system was affected, and the cancer proliferated.

Many writers of the past have made the connection between stress (or some other emotional problem) and cancer.

Two thousand years ago, Galen noted that women who were melancholy were much more susceptible to cancer than other females.

In 1701, Gendron, a British physician noted the effect of *"disasters of life as occasion much trouble and grief"* in the causation of cancer.

In the late 1700s, Burrows attributed cancer to *"the uneasy passions of the mind with which the patient is strongly affected for a long time."*

The early nineteenth century physician, Nunn, highlighted the emotional factors influencing the growth of breast tumours.

Historically, the development of cancer was attributed to emotional issues, but modern medicine cannot prove this.

Perhaps the physicians in the past knew their patients better. They relied more on a personal relationship with their patients rather than high tech, laboratory and radiological tests that are the norm today.

Modern doctors really do not get to know their patients. They rely mostly on pathology tests. They look at a piece of paper with numbers on it or a radiology report rather than the patient.

Cancer is very rare in primitive cultures, in fact, the more civilized a culture becomes, the more the rate of cancer increases.

The Tanchou doctrine

The French surgeon, Stanislas Tanchou (1791-1850), formulated a doctrine in 1843, which stated that the incidence of cancer (and insanity) increases in direct proportion to the civilization of the nation and its people. At that time, London had a cancer rate of 0.2 per thousand, while Paris had a rate of 0.8 per thousand. He proudly concluded that Paris is four times more civilized than London!

Since cancer is a **disease of civilization**, what is, or are, the causes? Firstly, there is the diet as we have been discussing, then there is the pollution. Then, perhaps it is the stress. Although stress is admittedly a vague term. Stress is not what is out there. Stress is how the person interprets what is out there.

Dai et al. (2020) showed that chronic stress does

promote cancer development.

The more civilized a nation and its people, the more pressures, laws, expectations, and responsibilities there are on the people.

Modern, civilized society does not tolerate the primitive, fight and flight reaction. There are no more sabre-toothed tigers but there are bosses, police, judges, parking inspectors, tax commissioners, various administrators, officials, etc.: the more civilized a society, the larger the number of people controlling you.

This leads to a whole host of emotional stresses. The fight or flight response is no longer appropriate or useful. Trying to suppress this primeval reflex can be very stressful and can lead to chronic disease, hypertension, diabetes, and cancer.

Hans Seyle in his studies of stress found that not all stress is bad; there is good stress or “eustress” as he called it. There is a system of checks and balances. The good stress can balance out the bad stress.

This idea of “good” and “bad”, positive, and negative, stimulating, and antagonistic is a very common concept found in nature. In any finely tuned mechanism, there are always opposing forces to ensure fine control.

The ancient Chinese had the concept of the *yin* and

the *yang* as represented in the familiar symbol.

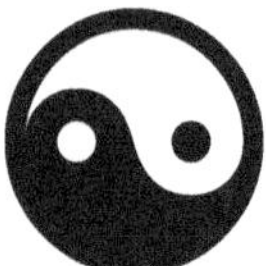

Black, white, though in balance. The white has a bit of black and the black has a bit of white. Opposite to each other but complementary and both are needed, in balance, for optimal health.

This can be seen in the autonomic nervous system, the sympathetic and the parasympathetic systems, opposite function to each other but both needed for balance and health. The same with hormones: they usually work in pairs, one stimulating and the other antagonistic, but both are needed in balance for optimal health.

Even the car has a brake and an accelerator. What sort of car would only have a brake, or only an accelerator? You need both but in balance.

There is good stress which can promote health. Consider planning for a holiday overseas. The planning, the purchase of tickets, organizing a passport, all stressful but a good stress.

Here we get back to the concept where a medically stable person deteriorates and dies soon after hearing of bad news or after the death of a loved one. Or conversely, people recovering from serious illness, without specific therapy but who were optimistic and not worried and not "stressed".

There are emotional aspects that are needed, things like faith, love, caring family and friends, a social support: these are all stress buffers. These have been shown to reduce the incidence of cancer as well as improving outcomes.

On the other hand, lack of faith, love and social support is cancer promoting.

Many cancer cures do rely on faith.

What sort of society do we live in?

A cold, unsporting, loveless society where relationships frequently break down and selfish, uncaring attitudes are common. It is no wonder cancer develops.

Sleep

In line with the earlier theme regarding lack of sleep and the development of MetS, cancer development is no different. Cancer can be prevented by getting adequate sleep. Earlier we have seen that the light/dark circadian rhythm is related to melatonin secretion. Melatonin is a powerful antioxidant and a lack of sleep, or a disrupted circadian rhythm can disrupt melatonin secretion predisposing to cancer development.

Many studies have shown a link between sleep disruption, disturbances of circadian rhythms (e.g., shift workers), excess artificial lighting at night and cancer (Filipski et al., 2002; Sephon & Spiegel, 2003; Pauley, 2004; Stevens, 2006).

Melatonin has been shown to be an effective adjuvant treatment to conventional cancer drugs (Talib, Alsayed, Abuawad, Daoud, & Mahmod, 2021).

Studies of blind women have shown them to have 36% less breast cancer than sighted women. This would support the melatonin hypothesis that increased night-time exposure to artificial light reduces melatonin levels, altering oestrogen secretion rates and upping risks for breast cancer. Blind women are unresponsive to light and have high melatonin production at night despite bright environmental night lighting (Kliukiene, Tynes,

& Andersen, 2001; Feychting, Osterlund, & Ahlbom, 1998).

So, a good idea is to sleep in the dark.

There may be other explanations: perhaps blind women do not go out as much, do not party as hard, have a different diet and life-style due to their blindness.

Exercise can reduce the risk of cancer. This is possibly tied in with weight loss, reducing IR and getting out into the sunshine.

As discussed above, there are a number of factors, diet and the carcinogens in today's environment, stress, the lack of exercise, the lack of sleep, the increased level of night illumination, all related to the modern lifestyle and therefore a cause of **death by civilization.**

OTHER MANIFESTATIONS OF METABOLIC SYNDROME

"The part can never be well unless the whole is well."
Plato (c427 – 348 BCE)

We have explored the "Deadly Quintet" of obesity, diabetes, cholesterol, hypertension, and cancer. These are all **diseases of civilization** caused mainly by the highly refined, sugar-laden diet, the lifestyle that is contradictory to our genetics, pollution, and almost as important, the stress in our society.

MetS has many other manifestations, with new ones being discovered continually. Some are not deadly, just annoying: others are much more serious, adding to **Death by Civilization**.

Here we are looking at conditions as varied as poly cystic ovary syndrome (PCOS), acne vulgaris, myopia, skin tags, acanthosis nigricans, early menarche, increased stature, male vertex balding, fatty liver, gallstones, sleep apnoea and Alzheimer's disease. I will only discuss some of these. Of course, dealing with the underlying metabolism is a major part of treating these conditions.

The above list is a group of varying conditions that seemingly are unrelated, although there are some common underlying characteristics. There is enhanced or unregulated growth, such as we have already seen with cancer, but which also happens with skin tags, myopia, and increased stature.

Excess testosterone production caused by hyperinsulinaemia has a role in the hormone imbalances found in PCOS. Fat storage caused by insulin can lead to fatty liver. Still others are related in ways, we are not sure how. However, all have some underlying association with IR and hyperinsulinaemia, the major **disease of civilization**.

Polycystic ovary syndrome (PCOS)

PCOS is a common disorder in women and can be defined as being caused by a hormonal imbalance with excess androgens. Symptoms of PCOS include irregular or no periods, acne, obesity, and excess hair growth. This disorder often prevents ovulation, leading to infertility. It is associated, perhaps even caused by IR.

The extreme form is the Stein-Leventhal syndrome but there is a spectrum which can range from just mild irregular periods to the full manifestation. Mild cases do not even have to have polycystic ovaries. So, any woman with any gynaecological problem can have a mild form of PCOS. It is important to treat the underlying metabolism first rather than simply treating any superficial manifestations.

Insulin inhibits the enzyme *aromatase,* which converts testosterone to oestrogen. With IR and hyperinsulinaemia, the pituitary signals the ovaries to make oestrogen. Since the testosterone cannot be converted, the brain detects that oestrogen is not being made and stimulates the ovaries even more. More testosterone is made but is not converted to oestrogen. Of course, in a female, increased levels of testosterone are not a good thing. Many of the symptoms of PCOS can be related to high testosterone levels.

As we have already seen, hyperinsulinaemia and IR are a part of the **diseases of civilization**, caused by the extremely highly refined, high sugar diet found in western society. PCOS can be helped by improving IR with a change in diet, supplements, and herbs, as well as increasing exercise and vitamin D.

In a large intervention study, Berrino et al. (2001) demonstrated that diets rich in low-glycaemic foods reduced serum testosterone and fasting glucose, while improving insulin metabolism and increasing SHBG. This study did not specifically look at PCOS, it just looked at the hormonal changes related to diet.

PCOS can lead to infertility. If the population is becoming more and more insulin resistant, then fertility is compromised. This certainly would lead to increasing difficulties with reproducing and ultimately, the worst scenario, to extinction.

According to the World Health Organisation (WHO), presently, 1 in 6 (17.5% of adults) worldwide has fertility issues.

(https://www.who.int/news/item/04-04-2023-1-in-6-people-globally-affected-by-infertility - Accessed 3 October 2023)

While we are on the topic of infertility, pollution needs to be mentioned. Many of these pollutants are chemicals that are xenoestrogens: chemicals that have hormonal/oestrogenic actions. They have a devastating effect on the body's hormonal system, either as a hormonal blocker or as a hormonal mimicker. They are producing an epidemic of infertility in women, low sperm counts in men, cancers of the genital tract in women (cancer of breast, cervix, uterus) and men (prostate, testes), as well as the feminisation of men.

This will have an impact on future generations. Sperm count has declined by 50% over the last 40 years and is most likely due to xenoestrogens (Levine et al., 2017; Rozati, Reddy, Reddanna, & Mujtaba, 2002; Sharpe & Skakkebaek, 1993).

Males have the potential to be feminised *in utero* due to the high level of xenoestrogens (Gonsioroski, Mourikes, & Flaws, 2020).

If this trend continues, our whole species could become extinct.

Mann, Shiff, and Patel (2020) wrote that *"Several retrospective and basic science studies have shown possible links for this decline in sperm parameters such as obesity, diet, and environmental toxins."*

Female babies are born with a total complement of ova in their ovaries, therefore any damage to ovaries *in utero* by xenoestrogens and other chemicals can have long lasting effects, affecting even the next generation (Woodruff & Walker 2008).

Male genital abnormalities are occurring in increasing numbers; the rate of testicular cancer in the USA and Europe has greatly increased in the past 50 years, and the occurrence of other male genital abnormalities such as, undescended testes, and hypospadias also greatly increased between the 1940s and the 1970s (Sengupta, 2014).

What could have a greater impact on our species than increasing infertility? Surely this would be included in **Death by Civilization.**

Alzheimer's disease

Alzheimer's disease (AD) is a neurodegenerative disease characterized by progressive cognitive degeneration, which includes loss of memory, intellectual deterioration with loss of language, recognition, and skilled movements. AD is the most common form of dementia.

This condition is becoming more and more common, and I do not have to elaborate on the impact it is having on our society. Caring for people with AD is having a huge impact on our society emotionally and financially, not just for the family and carers of these people but for society and the health care system in general.

More than 4.5 million in the USA are believed to have this condition and it is estimated there will be up to

13.2 million by 2050. If this is happening in the USA, the rest of the western world is not far behind.

In Australia, the cost of Alzheimer's disease is expected to rise by more than 70 per cent to around $26.6 billion over the next 20 years.

(https://www.dementia.org.au › about-us › media-centre › media-releases › 266-billion-cost-alzheimers - Accessed 18 November 2023)

This certainly can be classified as a **disease of civilization.**

Up until recently, no cause had been found, but newer studies are beginning to make the picture clearer. One of the basic characteristic histopathologic findings are amyloid plaques, composed of the amyloid A-beta peptides, and by aggregates of tau appearing as neurofibrillary tangles, neuritic plaques and neuronal threads. Tau is a microtubule-associated protein (MAP) that is an important component of the neurofibrillary tangles which is found in brain cells and is a hallmark of AD.

As far back as 1994, Razay and Wilcock noted a relationship between hyperinsulinaemia and AD. Patients with AD tend to have higher insulin levels and higher body mass index i.e. obesity.

AD, as previously noted, has been related to IR and has been referred to as type 3 diabetes. AD is “diabetes of the brain.”

Janoutová, Machaczka, Zatloukalová, and Janout (2022) concluded *“Because of similar molecular and cellular features among type 1 and type 2 diabetes and insulin resistance associated with memory deficit and cognitive decline, some researchers proposed the term "type 3 diabetes" for Alzheimer's disease.”*

Whitmer, Gunderson, Barrett-Connor, Quesenberry, and Yaffe (2005) noted that obesity in middle age increases the risk of future dementia independently of co-morbid conditions.

IR plays a role in the pathophysiology and clinical symptoms of AD (Watson & Craft, 2003).

Craft (2005) showed that insulin plays an important role in memory and other aspects of brain function. IR reduces insulin activity and reduces brain insulin levels and is associated with age-related memory impairment and AD.

Fishel et al. (2005) concluded that “*Moderate hyperinsulinemia can elevate inflammatory markers and Abeta42 in the periphery and the brain, thereby potentially increasing the risk of Alzheimer’s disease.”*

From CBS News (26 June 2007) "*New findings suggest that poorly controlled diabetes may lead to Alzheimer's disease. The worry is that today's mushrooming diabetes epidemic will become tomorrow's Alzheimer's epidemic, researchers said at the American Diabetes Association's 67th Annual Scientific Sessions, held June 22-26, 2007, in Chicago.*"

"*Craft (Professor Suzanne Craft, Professor of Psychiatry and Behavioural Science University of Seattle, Washington) has also found that the relatively high levels of insulin in people with type 2 diabetes may spur development of the amyloid protein that is present in the brains of Alzheimer's patients. High insulin levels may also trigger a cascade of potentially harmful chemical signals in the brain.*"

The modern western diet, which is low in omega 3, low in antioxidants and high in TFAs has been linked to the development of AD.

Contrast this to our ancestral diet, which was high in omega 3, high in antioxidants and virtually nil in TFAs.

One possible treatment of AD is the use of coconut oil. Coconut oil is composed of medium-chain fatty acids (MCFA) that are easily absorbed and converted in the liver to ketones which are an alternative energy source for the brain. Since IR reduces glucose entry into the brain cells, the ketones bypass the IR giving the brain cells an alternate source of energy (Fernando et al., 2015).

Does this work?

In a study, de la Rubia Ortí et al. (2017) concluded that coconut oil improves cognitive abilities of AD patients. The researchers followed up with a pilot study (de la Rubia Ortí et al., 2018). They concluded that *"The isocaloric coconut oil enriched Mediterranean diet seems to improve cognitive functions in patients with AD..."*

Another way is by adopting a "ketogenic diet". This is a high fat, low carbohydrate diet that puts the body into ketosis. These ketones can supply an alternate energy source to the brain cells as well as possibly helping to reduce the accumulation of amyloid plaques while reducing amyloid β toxicity (Broom, Shaw, & Rucklidge, 2019).

Another aspect is exercise.

Exercise was a regular part of our ancestral lifestyle. Unfortunately, in this modern world, exercise has become a very small part. Exercise can help to prevent dementia, AD or otherwise. Larson et al. (2006) concluded that regular exercise is associated with a delay in onset of dementia and AD, further supporting its value for elderly persons.

Many of these studies I have quoted are over 15 years old. Has the thinking about AD and MetS changed?

The newest study found is from 2023, and the thinking has not changed.

"AD is highly associated with metabolic syndrome, defined as the combination of hypertension, hyperlipidemia, obesity and type 2 diabetes mellitus (T2DM)." "It has been suggested that the mechanism linking both conditions is insulin resistance." "Insulin desensitization, therefore, could impact normal brain function increasing the risk of developing neurodegenerative disorders in later life" (Ezkurdia, Ramírez, & Solas, 2023).

Although not specific for AD, many people diagnosed with dementia have been found to be vitamin D deficient: is this a chicken or egg situation? Vitamin D deficiency has been found in many who reside in aged care facilities. It has been implicated in depression, psychiatric illness, and dementia. Of course, many residents in aged care facilities with dementia, or depression, or other mental illnesses, do not go out into the sun, so it could be a result rather than a cause.

Many with dementia and cognitive declinc have been found to have low vitamin D levels (Navale, Mulugeta, Zhou, Llewellyn, & Hyppönen, 2022).

The big question to ask is "Does supplementing vitamin D improve this mental decline?"

There is evidence that in some situations, (e.g. vitamin D deficiency) vitamin D may improve mental decline. Ghahremani et al. (2023) concluded that *"Across all formulations, vitamin D exposure was associated with significantly longer dementia-free survival and lower dementia incidence rate than no exposure (hazard ratio = 0.60, 95% confidence interval: 0.55–0.65). The effect of vitamin D on incidence rate differed significantly across the strata of sex, cognitive status, and APOE ε4 status."*

Therefore, if you do find a low vitamin D level in an elderly person, supplement and/or advise more sun exposure, at least it will help their bones and their depression, and you may be surprised at their improvement in mental functioning.

Prevention is better than cure. Supplement early before dementia develops.

So, the basic underlying metabolic disorder that this book is all about, IR and related hyperinsulinaemia, is possibly a cause of AD. We do know that IR and hyperinsulinaemia are becoming more and more prevalent. This will definitely increase the incidence of AD. If AD gets worse, then a larger and larger proportion of the population will develop dementia and be unable to function properly. This certainly fits into the category of **disease of civilization** and therefore can be included in **Death by Civilization.**

Fatty liver

The most common liver disease in western countries is the "fatty liver", where fat is deposited into the liver cells, causing liver cell enlargement, liver damage and liver dysfunction. It can range from sub-clinical, with little or no symptoms to severe, with profound complications. Severe cases can lead to inflammation of the liver and eventual fibrosis, which is called cirrhosis.

The most common causes are related to lifestyle, notably alcohol and diet.

Alcohol is a liver poison. I do not think more needs to be said. Avoid or minimise alcohol intake and the liver will recover.

Even though alcohol abuse is rife, a more common cause of fatty liver exists, and that is the western diet.

The fatty liver has been described as the hepatic manifestation of MetS (Marchesini, Marzocchi, Agostini, & Bugianesi, 2005). This is referred to as non-alcoholic fatty liver disease (NAFLD).

MetS is the basis of most of the diseases of western civilization; the high carbohydrate diet is a major cause, with the epigenetic changes that can affect the coming generations. Highly refined foods, such as sugars and grains, especially the refined flour, breads, cereals, and noodles all raise serum insulin and convert everything to fat. Not only do our abdomens get fat but so does the liver.

Many have blamed the fat in the diet. It *seems* logical that eating fat would cause fatty liver, but the evidence is scant. Eating fat *per se* does not cause fatty liver. It is not the fat in the diet but the carbohydrates. Since fatty liver is a manifestation of MetS, this tells us that the main culprits are the sugars and carbohydrates. In fact, a higher fat intake can protect the liver.

Solga et al. (2004) showed that a higher fat intake was associated with significantly lower odds of inflammation, while a high carbohydrate diet was associated with significantly *higher* odds of inflammation. The study concluded that the present dietary recommendations (i.e., low fat, high carbohydrate diet) may worsen NAFLD.

Gallstones

The most common problem with the gallbladder is the formation of gallstones.

Gallstones are clumps of solid material that form in the gallbladder. Eighty percent are made from cholesterol and the remaining 20% are pigment stones consisting of calcium and bilirubin. Gallstones vary in size and number, ranging in size from a grain of sand to a golf ball. In some cases, only one stone develops, and they tend to be large, or they are multiple and small.

It is not a new disease: gallstones were found in the mummy of the Egyptian princess Amer who lived around approximately 1500 BCE (Ellis, 2019).

What is different in these modern times is the *frequency* of the disease. Various studies have shown a high prevalence of gallstones: 10.5% in women and 6.5% in men. This equates to approximately 20 million people in the USA.

Despite this high frequency, luckily, a large proportion (84.9% of women and 87.0% of men) are "silent" i.e. asymptomatic. They are only discovered incidentally while investigating something else. Silent gallstones do not need to be treated.

> *"If it ain't broke, don't fix it!"*
> **Thomas Bertram Lance (1931-2013)**

In line with the theme of this book, where I am linking IR and hyperinsulinaemia to **diseases of civilization**, it should not surprise you that even gallstones are a manifestation of MetS.

Hyperinsulinaemia may play an important role in the aetiology of gallstones even in individuals without diabetes and with normal serum glucose levels (Misciagna, Guerra, Di Leo, Correale, & Trevisan, 2000).

Chen et al. (2012) concluded that *"GSD (gall stone disease) appears to be strongly associated with MetS, and the more the components of MetS, the higher the prevalence of GSD."*

Sleep apnoea (SA)

Sleep apnoea (SA) is a sleep disorder where breathing is interrupted during sleep. The person, generally male and obese, tends to snore loudly and experiences temporary stoppage of breathing in-between to varying degrees. The person is asleep and does not necessarily wake up. Generally, it is the partner who notices the temporary cessation of breathing. The person, although asleep all night, generally has a poor quality of sleep, and tends to get very tired during the day. People have fallen asleep at work and while driving, which, obviously, can be very dangerous.

There is a strong relationship between SA, MetS and IR (Peled et al., 2007; Vgontzas, Bixler, & Chrousos, 2005).

The strongest risk factor is obesity, although there is a two-way relationship. SA affects 17% of the total population and 40-70% of the obese population (Framnes & Arble, 2018). Obesity is a risk factor for SA, but also SA can lead to more obesity. As we have seen, MetS can lead to obesity and SA can make obesity worse. SA can also aggravate MetS, so it is a bidirectional process.

An interesting question is – which came first? In most cases, it is the obesity that comes first; 58% of moderate to severe SA is due to obesity, however there are other factors including age, male gender, perimenopause, or menopause in women and craniofacial abnormalities (Hamilton & Joosten, 2017).

The episodes of intermittent hypoxia can cause inflammation, but also inflammation can cause SA. Which came first?

MetS is known to cause inflammation. Gaines et al. (2017) demonstrated inflammation from fat tissue precedes the development of SA. MetS is known to produce obesity and inflammation.

Can SA be treated with anti-inflammatory medications or lifestyle? Melaku et al. (2022) showed that a higher quality and anti-inflammatory diet and an overall healthy lifestyle can reduce SA risk. We have already discussed anti-inflammatory foods.

Gala and Seaman (2011) discussed a case where a lifestyle modification resolved SA to the extent the continuous positive airway pressure (CPAP) machine was not needed. This included a "low inflammation diet", weight loss, and exercise. The patient has kept well during a seven year follow up.

Theoretically, anti-inflammatory agents, such as curcumin, fish oil, MC, etc., can reduce the inflammation and help to treat SA, but there is little published evidence. However, a study of the Chinese traditional formula *Jiawei Di Tan Tang* was shown to attenuate oxidative stress and inflammatory responses in patients with SA and may relieve clinical symptoms

(Chen, Lin, Hong, Ye & Lin, 2016).

SA has been shown to increase risk of heart attack and diabetes. The smart ones that have read the book so far will realize that SA does not necessarily cause diabetes and heart attacks, but it is the underlying metabolism that causes both. Deal with the underlying metabolism and the sleep apnoea and the risk of heart attack and diabetes will reduce.

Treatment for sleep apnoea generally, is lifestyle changes, especially losing weight. Conventional treatment is with a continuous positive airway pressure (CPAP) machine. The people must sleep with a mask attached to the machine, and it forces air into the lungs when the person is not breathing. This of course only treats the symptoms but not the underlying problem.

From my clinical experience, when treating obese or diabetic patients with a high protein and low carbohydrate diet, as well as the nutrients, and herbs discussed, and even before there is significant weight loss, they make the spontaneous comment that they are sleeping better.

Osteoporosis

Osteoporosis is a condition where there is a

reduced mass of bone, leading to an increased predisposition to fractures.

Osteoporosis is a **disease of civilization**. People can die from osteoporosis; so therefore, it can be included in **Death by Civilization**.

The incidence is huge: osteoporosis accounts for 8.9 million fractures worldwide annually. Incidence is 6.3% of men and 21% of women over age 50-years. Hip fractures are possibly the worst fractures with a mortality rate of 20-24% after the first hip fracture. There is also a greater risk of dying in the five years after the fracture with 20% dying in the first year.

(https://www.osteoporosis.foundation › facts-statistics - Accessed 3 September 2023)

Despite what the mainstream doctors say, osteoporosis is not a disease: it is a symptom. A symptom of a faulty lifestyle. Although not strictly related to MetS, there are connections. We all lose bone as we age: osteoporosis is an exaggerated bone loss. Osteoporosis is not necessarily a condition of reduced calcium (Ca) intake but rather a condition of increased Ca loss. We have been led to believe that osteoporosis is solely a condition of Ca deficiency. This idea was implanted into our minds by clever advertisements so that dairy products and Ca tablets can be sold to "increase Ca levels."

Ca is not the full answer. There are many other factors which include diet, exercise, vitamin D, Mg, and trace minerals.

The level of bone mass is dependent on the peak bone mass (PBM) which is achieved in women in their early 20s and in men in their late 20s. Generally, men achieve a higher PBM than women: this is why osteoporosis is a bigger problem for women. The higher the PBM the less chance of osteoporosis with age.

PBM is achieved by exercise, good nutrition, and plenty of vitamin D.

Das, Crocombe, McGrath, Berry, and Mughal (2006) showed that a great proportion (70%) of British female teenagers are vitamin D deficient, which could increase the burden of osteoporosis in the future by not maximising their PBM.

Osteoporosis has a hereditary component. This is due to genetic abnormalities in the vitamin D receptor. This hereditary form does not increase bone loss *per se* but produces osteoporosis by preventing the attainment of maximum PBM.

Many teenagers do not eat healthily, nor do they exercise as much. This will all add to the burden of osteoporosis in the future.

There is a steady decrease in bone mass as we age. Obviously if we start with a higher PBM, there will be greater bone remaining later in life.

Another important issue is the rate of bone loss. There is a steady loss, approximately 1-3% after the menopause. However, there are factors that can increase this rate of loss. Factors such as,

- diet: high sugar and refined carbohydrates.
- lifestyle: reduced exercise and reduced sun exposure.
- habits: such as smoking, alcohol, and caffeine consumption.

Rhee et al, (2022) showed that there is a high correlation between MetS and osteoporosis in obese males and in obese postmenopausal women.

As we have already seen, the western diet is high in sugar and refined carbohydrates which leads to hyperinsulinaemia and IR, which results in Mg deficiency. This point is important because Mg is essential to Ca metabolism.

Mg is involved in:

- Ca absorption, especially active Ca transportation,
- formation of active vitamin D.
- integrity of bone crystal formation.
- binding of Ca to tooth enamel.

There is some evidence that the development of osteoporosis may not necessarily be due to a lack of Ca but primarily a Mg deficiency (Rondanelli et al., 2021).

With the epidemic of MetS, there is also an epidemic of Mg deficiency, which can contribute to the high incidence of osteoporosis.

Sojka and Weaver (1995) gave Mg supplements (average dose 250 mg/day) to a group of menopausal women for 2 years. The results showed a reduction in fractures as well as significant increase in bone density.

As I have mentioned many times, we eat too much sugar, and this influences our insulin levels. Sugar and insulin influence our bones. A high sugar diet has been shown to increase urinary Ca excretion.

"The effects of sucrose on urinary calcium are consistent with the hypothesis that insulin inhibits renal calcium reabsorption"

(Holl & Allen, 1987).

I have written much about soft drink consumption. Americans are huge soft drink consumers. The sugar and the phosphorus, in, especially cola drinks, are major contributors to osteoporosis (Tucker, et al., 2006; Fernando, Martha, & Evangelina,1999; DiNicolantonio, Mehta, Zaman, & O'Keefe, 2018).

Western habits such as smoking, caffeine, and alcohol drinking increase bone loss, although small doses of alcohol seem to be protective (Ilich, Brownbill, Tamborini, & Crncevic-Orlic, 2002).

While small doses of alcohol may have been shown to be protective, Cheraghi et al. (2019) showed that high doses (greater than two standard drinks daily) were associated with higher levels of osteoporosis.

Also note, those who drink lots of alcohol tend to stagger and fall, which will certainly add to the incidence of fractures.

Kemmler, Engelke, Weineck, Hensen, and Kalender (2003) demonstrated that exercise is needed to increase bone density, while not exercising reduces bone density.

Our paleolithic ancestors had better, stronger bones due to their increased workload. Bone strength started to decline when humans moved away from hunting and gathering and turned to agriculture. Ryan and Shaw (2015) showed that modern human skeletons are weaker and lighter due to decreased biomechanical loading.

Our current lifestyle involves sitting in the car, sitting behind a computer screen, sitting in front of the TV; humans were not designed to be inactive!

If you don't use it, you lose it!

....

"That which is used - develops. That which is not used wastes away."

Hippocrates (c460-c370 BCE)

Excess protein consumption has been implicated in osteoporosis, although this has to some extent been disproved. Our species evolved as a hunter-gatherer with a diet high in protein and fat. Evolution would not have allowed a high protein diet to cause osteoporosis.

The initial studies that showed Ca loss with high protein intake were done using isolated, fractionated amino acids from milk or eggs. However, Spencer, Kramer, DeBartolo, Norris, and Osis (1983) showed that when protein is given as meat, subjects do not show any increase in Ca excreted, or any significant change in serum Ca, and it does not lead to Ca loss, even over a long period.

Tsagari (2020) concluded that *"Current evidence shows no adverse effects of higher protein intakes."*

Mainstream medicine is fanatical about supplementing Ca: but how good is Ca on its own? Many trace minerals are also needed. Ca on its own is relatively useless and possibly dangerous. Also note that Ca on its own can be deposited in areas other than bone.

Strause, Saltman, Smith, Bracker, and Andon (1994) compared four groups of post-menopausal women over a 2-year period. The four groups were given various supplements,

1) Placebo.
2) Ca supplementation 1,000 mg daily.
3) Ca 1,000 mg plus Zn 15 mg plus manganese 5 mg plus copper 2.5 mg daily.
4) The above trace minerals only.

The best group i.e. the least bone loss, was the Ca

plus trace minerals group.

Boron (B) is particularly important for women because it is involved in the metabolism of Ca, Mg, and oestrogen. Low levels of B upset Ca metabolism, allowing Ca to be stripped more easily from the bones. Nielsen, Hunt, Mullen, and Hunt (1987) showed that a supplement of B (3 mg) improved Ca and Mg metabolism.

Fluoride (F)

There is a "pollutant", which is legally put into the drinking water: fluoride (F). This influences bone metabolism. F treatment was used to treat osteoporosis because it made the bones on x-rays look stronger (made the bones look whiter on the x-ray) but the bone became more brittle and could shatter more easily. Helte et al. (2021) showed that F can increase bone mineral density (BMD) but paradoxically, also increase bone fragility, therefore fracture more easily.

F can cause more fractures. Li et al. (2001) showed that there is an increased incidence of hip fracture in elderly people exposed to fluoridated water.

F can also affect intellectual development of babies.

Grandjean (2019) wrote that *"The recent epidemiological results support the notion that elevated fluoride intake during early development can result in IQ deficits that may be considerable."*

Till and Green (2021) authored an interesting paper, *"Controversy: The evolving science of fluoride: when new evidence doesn't conform with existing beliefs."* They wrote that the health authorities have declared that F is "safe and effective" - where have I heard this before? Rather than re-evaluate the earlier findings, any new evidence that goes against the established beliefs is ignored. Unfortunately, this can be applied to many things, not just fluoride.

So, we can see that osteoporosis is a **disease of civilization**. It is related to what we eat and how we live our lives. Osteoporosis is a part of **Death by Civilization.**

Acne vulgaris

Acne vulgaris is a common skin condition caused by androgen elevated sebum production, abnormal keratinization, bacterial colonisation, and inflammation.

Bungau et al. (2023) discussed the link between acne and MetS. The cause and severity of acne may be influenced by hyperinsulinaemia and IR (Hasrat & Al-Yassen, 2023).

Improving the diet can be very beneficial in the treatment of acne. This includes avoiding certain foods such as milk and chocolate and increasing foods with a high omega 3 content. Omega 3 fatty acids suppress inflammatory cytokines (Bungau et al., 2022).

A diet of high GI foods can trigger acne, while a diet with a low GI shows reduced acne (Conforti et al., 2022).

The Australian Women's Weekly magazine, in conjunction with the Australasian College of Dermatologists and the RMIT university, have published a booklet – *The Teenage Anti-Acne Diet* (available on-line). The diet is basically a higher protein, low GI, which includes low sugar, low processed foods, and low junk food intakes. This is in line with the diet/eating pattern that I have suggested throughout this book.

Acne is a **disease of civilization**, though not necessarily a **Death by Civilization.**

However, severe acne can lead to facial scarring which can have a lasting psychological impact: the face is visible to all and therefore can have a significant effect on a person's self-worth, self-esteem, and social standing. This can lead to anxiety and depression and can be quite significant, possibly even leading to suicide.

To make things worse, depression and IR are related, as we shall discuss in the next chapter.

Therefore, prevention is very important; deal with the acne early to prevent the scarring.

BEHAVIOUR and MENTAL HEALTH

The Tanchou Doctrine *(1843): the incidence of cancer* ***and insanity*** increases *in direct proportion to the civilization of the nation and its people.*
Stanislas Tanchou (1791-1850)

What is happening to today's society? Mental health issues are becoming more and more prominent. This is not hard to see. The whole world is going crazy! Is this a sign that the Tanchou Doctrine is valid?

Behaviour and mental health are related to:

- what we eat,
- the stresses we are subjected to in our society,
- modern lifestyle,
- the gut microbiome,
- lack of sleep,

- the chemical pollutants, and
- even drugs used by doctors to deal with some of these conditions.

Mental ill-health is definitely a **disease of civilization.**

The effect of diet and nutrition on heart disease or diabetes is generally well accepted and recognized, however, the effect of diet and nutrition on the mind has not been accepted (yet) to the same degree.

How can a modern, technologically advanced society function if a large proportion of the population has a disordered brain function? How can the society flourish when crime is rife, the children are aggressive and violent, when mental disorders are steadily increasing, when rates of dementia are growing, and when rates of autism and attention deficit hyperactivity disorder (ADHD) are skyrocketing?

How can a society survive when a large portion of the population is being drugged by mind-altering pharmaceuticals?

These are **diseases of civilization.**

These do impact on **Death by Civilization.**

The fabric of our society is being torn apart by a growing number of mental health issues in our children and even the adults. Some of these problems are real, others are not. Some diagnoses are invented by drug companies to make people believe they are "sick" and need "treatment". Some are just normal emotions being made into diseases and "treated" with drugs.

Depression

Depression is an all-too-common disorder in today's society.

The risk of developing a major depressive disorder is double if there is IR compared to someone who does not have IR (Watson et al., 2021).

One reason for this is to do with tryptophan metabolism. Tryptophan is an essential amino acid (meaning the body cannot manufacture it) and is the precursor of the neurotransmitter serotonin which is related to depression.

Tryptophan is obtained solely through diet, and the overall amount of tryptophan in food is quite low (approximately 1%), so it can be difficult to obtain adequate amounts through food intake. This would be aggravated by a low protein diet. Good sources of tryptophan include meat of any sort, fish, firm tofu, edamame, milk, squash and pumpkin seeds and eggs.

The absorption through the BBB can be low due to competition with other amino acids. However, insulin pushes many of the other large neutral amino acids into peripheral cells, and this gives tryptophan an easier passage into the brain through the BBB (Spring, 1984). IR would interfere with tryptophan passage through the BBB. Insulin is known to have an antidepressant effect. Therefore, IR would have an opposite effect (Zou, Sun, Yang, Li, & Cui, 2020).

Once tryptophan enters the brain, carbohydrates/insulin remain the main stimulant for production of serotonin. The need for carbohydrates, therefore insulin, for serotonin production may explain why depressed people eat more carbs and why junk foods are so popular; people reach out for refined sugar-laden foods and not the broccoli! This is a form of self-medication. Conversely, this craving for "feel good foods" may make the situation worse, as these foods are high in sugar and, as we have previously discussed, can aggravate the IR.

Tryptophan supplementation can be very useful in treating mental health issues. However, one issue with tryptophan supplementation is that there is a potential that tryptophan can go down other pathways and away from the serotonin pathway. This can be avoided by supplementing 5 hydroxytryptophan (5HTP). 5HTP is the second step in the serotonin pathway and cannot be reversed.

Tryptophan can be metabolised in three ways:

1. the serotonin pathway: tryptophan → 5 HTP → serotonin → melatonin.

2. the kynurenine pathway. This pathway, which accounts for over 90% of the tryptophan, can produce essential metabolites such as nicotinamide adenine dinucleotide (NAD^+) which is important for energy production, and niacin (vitamin B3). There are, however, negative metabolites such as kynurenine, kynurenic acid, and quinolinic acid which develop when the pathways are affected; this may play an important role in the pathophysiology of irritable bowel syndrome (IBS), Alzheimer's disease (AD), Parkinson's disease (PD), Huntington's disease (HD), schizophrenia, AIDS-dementia complex, depression, epilepsy, and the aging process.

The kynurenine/serotonin pathway isn't just in the brain but also in the gut. Therefore, gut issues may develop, such as IBS, gut motility issues and Vagus nerve stimulation. The gut microbiota also influences the tryptophan/kynurenine pathways.

3. the indole pathway. Indole and its metabolites have an anti-inflammatory action in intestinal cells and macrophages, as well as contributing to maintaining the biological barrier of the gut. Indoles improve intestinal health in such conditions as IBD, haemorrhagic colitis, and bowel cancer. This pathway is largely associated with the gut microbiota.

Another aspect of IR, as we have discussed earlier, is inflammation. Inflammation induces enzymes that push tryptophan down the kynurenine pathway, therefore reducing the pathway to serotonin production.

Stress also has a similar unbalancing effect on the kynurenine/serotonin pathways. Stress is a big issue in today's world as has been discussed previously.

Inflammation and stress are related to depression.

The gut microbiome plays a role here. There is a direct influence of the gut microbiota on serotonergic networks (Correia & Vale, 2022).

As you can see, the gut and the microbiota have a

major role in mental health, therefore, keep your gut and microbiome happy.

How does IR relate to this? The dysregulation of the tryptophan-kynurenine pathway is one of the mechanisms of IR (Oxenkrug, 2013).

Many psychiatric illnesses are associated with MetS. This does not necessarily mean that MetS causes psychiatric illness, but it can complicate the course of the disease. This may also develop into a two-way process, as MetS does impact brain function in various ways, including impaired vascular reactivity, neuroinflammation, oxidative stress, and abnormal brain lipid metabolism. This can possibly aggravate psychiatric illness (Yates, Sweat, Yau, Turchiano, & Convit, 2012).

> *"If you are in a bad mood, go for a walk. If you are still in a bad mood, go for another walk."*
> **Hippocrates (c460-c370 BCE)**

Other aspects

Behavioural problems in children are getting worse. Of course, some behavioural issues may be the result of lack of discipline, boredom, alienation, bullying, domestic violence at home, and violent films, and videogames, but equally some are related to diet. The growing incidence of crime, violence, vandalism, truancy, uncontrollable behaviour, lack of respect for others, and so on are becoming significant problems.

If these trends continue, a great majority of the population will be mentally affected. Who will be in charge? Will there be a small number of individuals with "normal" cognitive function who run the show and while a great majority does not have the mental capacity to pose any opposition? What if the leaders are mentally deranged?

Is this already happening?

A report titled, "*Feeding Minds; The impact of food on mental health*" was released by the Mental Health Foundation in the UK in 2007.

(https://www.bl.uk › collection-items › feeding-minds-the-impact-of-food-on-mental-health - Accessed 4 September 2023)

The report comments on the fact that mental health problems are growing at an ever-increasing rate. In the UK, the yearly cost for mental health is approaching £100 billion a year. Diet and nutrition factors are not generally recognized by mainstream medicine, yet it is possibly one of the major factors that can reduce and prevent much suffering.

As we have seen so far, the human diet has altered greatly over the past few thousand years and the change has been even greater in the last hundred years or so.

From a very basic point of view, our moods, our behaviour, our perception are all based on the optimal functioning of our brain. Feed the brain well and it will function well.

Our brain is like a Ferrari and needs proper fuel. Kerosene and diesel are good fuels but if we try to fuel the Ferrari with kerosene, or diesel, it will not work to its maximal efficiency or ability… or perhaps at all!

The brain is not being fuelled optimally. As mentioned above, the way we eat, as well as what we eat, has changed dramatically over the last 50-100 years. This theme has already been discussed earlier: the focus of this chapter is the effect of food and pollution on the functioning of the brain.

There have been big changes in the food we eat, not just to the types of food we eat, but also in the actual content of macronutrients and micronutrients in the food. There have also been changes in the farming methods and the use of chemicals, both in agriculture (pesticides, weedicide, artificial fertilizers) to chemicals being deliberately added, such as colours, flavours, and preservatives.

Research scientists at the UK's Asthma & Allergy Research Centre, working on behalf of the Food Standards Agency, concluded that *'significant changes in children's hyperactive behaviour could be produced by the removal of colourings and additives from their diet'.*

This is confirmed by McCann et al. (2007) who concluded that *"Artificial colours or a sodium benzoate preservative (or both) in the diet results in increased hyperactivity in 3-year-old and 8/9-year-old children in the general population."*

We are eating much less fresh produce and eating increasingly more processed foods. These foods are so highly processed that they have been referred to as "ultra-processed" foods, and they contain added sugars and colours, flavours, and preservatives, with very little fibre and nutrition. It has been estimated that the average person in the UK and other western societies consumes over four kilograms of additives every year. These ultra-processed foods with all the additives not only cause physical health issues such as obesity, cardiovascular disease, MetS, (as we have already discussed) but they also influence our mental health and our behaviour by altering brain function (Srour & Touvier, 2021).

There is a new discipline called "nutritional psychiatry". It involves looking at the mood-food connection and is largely modulated by the gut microbiome; the "gut-brain" connection (Naidoo, 2019).

The use of prebiotics, probiotics, and a gut-healthy diet have been shown to have a positive effect on mental health and psychological function (Ansari, Pourjafar, Tabrizi, & Homayouni, 2020).

"... increasing evidence indicates a strong association between a poor diet and the exacerbation of mood disorders, including anxiety and depression, as well as other neuropsychiatric conditions" (Adan et al., 2019).

Twenty percent of our brain is made up of essential fatty acids (EFA), notably omega 3 and 6. We have already seen that the optimal ratio of omega 3 to 6 is a one-to-one ratio, i.e. equal parts. Our species evolved eating foods with this ratio, it is what our ancestors ate. We are now eating an unbalanced ratio; too much omega 6. The relative lack of omega 3 (or excess omega 6) has been implicated in several mental health problems such as deression, anxiety, ADD, dementia, including AD, as well as problems with concentration and memory. This situation is exacerbated by the inclusion of TFAs in our diet.

Schizophrenia has been shown to be associated with lower serum omega 3 fatty acids (Jones et al., 2021).

The neurotransmitters, the messengers that communicate between the brain cells are made up of amino acids derived from the diet. A low protein diet cannot supply the raw materials needed to make the neurotransmitters. Minerals, such as Zn, Mg, and vitamins such as vitamin B6, B12, and folate are essential for proper brain function. These nutrients come from our diet, but our eating habits have changed; the amount of these nutrients have decreased. Over the last sixty years, there has been a 34% decline in vegetable consumption in the UK. Only 13% of men and 15% of women are eating the recommended five portions of fruit and vegetable per day. There has been a 59% decrease in fish consumption over the last sixty years. Instead of eating a healthy diet, more and more young people are eating a diet of ultra-processed foods.

The Mental Health Foundation report noted that, *"Nearly two thirds of those who do not report daily mental health problems eat fresh fruit or fruit juice every day, compared with less than half of those who do report daily mental health problems. This pattern is similar for fresh vegetables and salad." "Those who report some level of mental health problem also eat fewer healthy foods (fresh fruit and vegetables, organic foods and meals made from scratch) and more unhealthy foods (chips and crisps, chocolate, ready meals and takeaways)."*

Mental health is related to diet. Just look at what we are eating. One of the main culprits is sugar. Many parents can see that their children become "hyperactive" on sugar, yet mainstream doctors do not seem to, or want to accept this. They have done studies and they have found no relationship. The meta-analysis by Wolraich, Wilson, and White (1995) concluded *"The meta-analytic synthesis of the studies to date found that sugar does not affect the behavior or cognitive performance of children."*

Try telling this to parents who do see their children going ballistic on sugar. Try telling this to parents who see their children respond positively to dietary change.

However, it may not be just the sugar. Parents relate that their children go ballistic after attending a birthday party. Here the children are exposed not just to sugar, but colours, flavours, and preservatives. Also, the excitement of the party may contribute to these behaviours.

There have been studies where parents were told

that the child was given a high sugar load, and in fact, a placebo was given. The study concluded that it was largely a parental expectation that was the problem (Hoover & Milich, 1994).

Note that these studies were done in the 1990s.

Changes are afoot!

A study published in 2006 by Lien, Lien, Heyerdahl, Thoresen, and Bjertness looked at whether high levels of consumption of sugar-containing soft drinks were associated with mental distress, hyperactivity, and conduct problems among adolescents. The researchers concluded, *"High consumption levels of sugar-containing soft drinks were associated with mental health problems among adolescents even after adjustment for possible confounders."*

Suglia, Solnick, and Hemenway (2013) studied soft drink consumption in five-year-olds and found aggressive behaviour increased with the number of soft drink servings per day. Children who drank four or more servings a day were twice as likely to physically attack people and destroy other people's property compared to children who did not drink soft drinks.

Other than sugar, soft drinks contain highly processed ingredients such as aspartame, sodium benzoate, phosphoric acid, and citric acid. So, which is it that is affecting the behaviour?

Of course, the American Beverage Association (ABA) slammed this study.

A study by Moore, Carter, and van Goozen (2009) showed that excess consumption of confectionery at age ten predicts convictions for violence in adulthood.

The level of intake of sugary drinks is very high indeed.

Sugar can cause behavioural problems as we have seen, as well as general health problems such as obesity and diabetes which is related to MetS, inflammation and dental caries/oral health.

Skallevold, Rokaya, Wongsirichat, and Rokaya, (2023) showed the interplay of oral health and mental disorders, such as depression, anxiety, bipolar disorder, schizophrenia, dementia, and alcohol and drug use disorders. This interplay involves dysregulated microbiome, translocated bacteria, and systemic inflammation.

Dental health must be included in the treatment of mental health problems. Unfortunately, dental services are not cheap, and many cannot afford to have regular dental treatments. The government dental health services have long waiting lists, and the dental pathology will get much worse while waiting for treatment.

What other foods cause behavioural problems?

Two of the staple foods are perhaps the worst offenders. These foods have already been mentioned many times in this book: grains and dairy, specifically gluten and casein.

One of the theories of autism is the opioid excess theory, which is where peptides of exogenous origin affect neurotransmission in the brain. Tarnowska et al. (2023) wrote that the theory has *"neither been definitively confirmed nor disproved."*

These peptides have opioid activity and therefore have effects on perception, cognition, emotions, mood, and behaviour.

Exogenous opioid peptides come from the incomplete breakdown of certain foods, notably gluten and casein: grains and dairy. Due to poor digestive function, gluten and casein are improperly broken down and these peptides are absorbed, especially if there is a "leaky gut". These peptides have opioid activity that affects brain function.

This can be shown by examining urine of children with autism. If the urine is examined using high performance liquid chromatography (HPLC), various peaks of protein are found. In children with autism, one of these peaks corresponds to bovine-casomorphine which is not found in children without autism.

One of the assumptions is that these biologically active opioid peptides are absorbed and influence the brain. D'Eufemia et al. (1996) showed that children with autism have a "leaky gut" i.e. greater gut permeability, than children who do not have autism.

"Leaky gut" is a condition where there is an abnormality in the gut and more gut contents (toxins, peptides, etc.) which normally are denied entry, can enter the body.

Many children, whether they have autism or are simply badly behaved, do respond positively to a gluten free and dairy free diet. These foods should never have been introduced into the human diet in the first place. Dairy is good only for baby cows, and gluten has never been a part of the human diet until only relatively recently. I have been saying for a long time that cow's milk is only good for baby cows. However, cow's milk is very low in Mg, so that a calf must start to eat grass at 1-2 weeks of age to get adequate Mg.

As already mentioned, there are those who seem to tolerate dairy and grains. However, those who cannot are the ones who develop mood issues and gut complaints.

> *"What is food to one man is bitter poison to others."*
> **Lucretius (c99-c55 BCE)**

I have personally seen remarkable improvements in the behaviour of children, once they eliminate sugar, dairy, and gluten, from their diets.

Dairy seems to cause the most behavioural problems. These children are dairy intolerant, not necessarily dairy allergic. Mainstream doctors do not seem to understand the difference between dairy allergy and dairy intolerance. Dairy intolerance is a non-allergic response, therefore there is a negative result on dairy allergy testing. With food intolerances, the best way to diagnose, and treat, is firstly to eliminate, then re-challenge.

Many "hyperactive" children, children with ADD, "badly behaved" children may have a food allergy or intolerance, most commonly to dairy or gluten. Thankfully, newer studies are now recognizing the connection between behaviour and food.

Bateman et al. (2004) wrote that *"There is a general adverse effect of artificial food colouring and benzoate preservatives on the behaviour of 3 year old children which is detectable by parents but not by a simple clinic assessment."*

Breakey (1997) wrote that *"The research has shown that diet definitely affects some children. Rather than becoming simpler the issue has become demonstrably more complex. The range of suspect food items has broadened, and some non-food items are relevant. Symptoms which may change include those seen in attention deficit disorder (ADD) and attention deficit hyperactivity disorder (ADHD), sleep problems and physical symptoms, with later research emphasizing particularly changes in mood."*

The important point is that diet seems to affect only a sub-group of children, although we are not sure of the size of that sub-group (from my clinical experience, that group is significant, although I should mention that many do self-refer to me, so I do get a biased population).

On the other hand, some of these foods shouldn't be in the human diet anyway, so, let's eliminate them from all children.

Case Study: Dairy intolerance.

A mother rang me and requested that I refer her 15-year-old daughter to a psychiatrist because of her behaviour. She would be violent, moody, depressed, angry, and irritable and always yelling and totally uncontrollable. She never had a good word for anyone. She had left home and was also in the process of leaving school. She also had bad 'sinus' problems. I asked mother to bring her to me so we could get to the cause of her problem. Mother said that she was always difficult. Even as a baby she was crying, irritable, not sleeping, colicky and had eczema and asthma as well as recurrent infections requiring many courses of antibiotics. She was not breast fed. Since the problem started very early on in life, I thought that the cause could be a food intolerance. Dairy seemed to be the logical culprit. I advised her to have a 2-week dairy free diet. After 2 weeks she was a different person. She moved back home, started back at school, and became a 'normal person'. She continues to be 'good' only if she avoids dairy products.

Heavy metals (HMs)

We live on a polluted planet; this is nothing new. I have talked about HMs relating to other issues. HMs (and here I am NOT talking about the music, though that may influence behaviour in some) can influence brain function and therefore behaviour.

HMs are pollutants that can have multiple drastic effects on the human species. The list is long and varied: memory loss, increased allergic reactions, high blood pressure, depression, mood swings, irritability, poor concentration, aggressive behaviour, sleep issues, fatigue, speech disorders, high cholesterol, triglycerides, vascular occlusion, neuropathy, autoimmune diseases, and chronic fatigue. As you can see, some of the effects relate to topics discussed in previous chapters. Some relate to the topic at hand.

Acute excess exposure to HMs is dangerous but then chronic low-level exposure is more insidious and can also be just as dangerous.

The HMs I am referring to especially are Pb, Hg, Cd, and As.

These substances are found in nature but are generally locked away, prevented from doing us harm. However, with mining, mineral smelting, industrial pollution, and refining, many of these toxic metals are released into the environment, the water, the air and eventually end up in our bodies. We absorb these toxins, and they can accumulate in our bodies. HMs disrupt cellular enzyme systems by displacing and competing with the essential minerals such as Mg, Zn, and Se: this causes widespread disruption of nerve, brain, hormonal, and immune systems.

HMs, such as Hg and Pb seem to have a particular affinity to brain and nervous tissue and as such have a drastic effect on behaviour, cognition, memory, emotional lability, and produce other neurological problems. Children with autism have been found to have high levels of Hg, possibly due to the mercury-based preservative, thiomersal, used in the past in vaccines. Vaccines and/or Hg toxicity have been one of the theories offered to explain the recent increased incidence of autism, although now, the Hg has been mostly removed. This link is very controversial and mostly denied by mainstream doctors. However, Desoto and Hitlan (2007) reanalysed an earlier paper and have shown that there was error in the analysis of the data. They concluded that the data did show that there is a link between blood levels of Hg and autism.

Pb, in the past, was used in water pipes, was a component of paint and was also used in solder used for making tins for food storage, including baby formula. Pb toxicity of the central nervous system causes delayed development, diminished intelligence and altered behaviour, especially in children.

HMs have also been linked to criminal behaviour.

Needleman, McFarland, Ness, Fienberg, and Tobin (2002) concluded that *"Elevated body lead burdens, measured by bone lead concentrations, are associated with elevated risk for adjudicated delinquency."*

However, Beckley et al. (2018) did not show an association between lead and criminality. Their argument is that earlier studies were not confounded for socio-economic factors.

In a newer study, Wright et al. (2021) concluded that *"Childhood blood lead concentration prospectively predicted variation in adult arrests and arrests over the life-course, indicating lead absorption is implicated in the etiology of crime—especially in geographic areas where environmental sources of lead are more prevalent and concentrated."*

Treatment for HMs poisoning is chelation therapy, which I have already discussed.

HMs are pollutants from industry and mining. They have a drastic effect on our health and behaviour; they are a cause of **disease of civilization.**

There is a connection between diet, nutrition, and criminal behaviour.

Food intolerance is a factor in criminality. There is widespread recognition that hyperactivity in children is often followed by criminality. Trials have shown that many hyperactive children can be cured, or at least their behaviour modified, by dietary changes and, as such, criminality in later years can be prevented.

"Antisocial behaviour in prisons, including violence, are reduced by vitamins, minerals and essential fatty acids with similar implications for those eating poor diets in the community" (Gesch, Hammond, Hampson, Eves, & Crowder, 2002).

Schoenthaler and Bier (2000) showed that supplementing school children with vitamin and mineral supplements, compared to a placebo, reduced institutional violence and antisocial behaviour by almost half.

We have already looked at the connection between suicide, criminal behaviour, and low cholesterol levels. Low blood cholesterol is associated with aggression and antisocial behaviour. People whose cholesterol levels were low were significantly more antisocial compared to others whose cholesterol was normal or higher.

Fiedorwicz and Haynes (2010) pose the question whether it is the low cholesterol that leads to depression and suicide or is it the depression that changes diet and lifestyle which can cause the low cholesterol?

Engelberg (1992) showed that low cholesterol levels decrease the number of serotonin receptors in the brain, which may contribute to a decrease in brain serotonin activity, leading to a poorer suppression of aggressive behaviour.

Segoviano-Mendoza et al. (2018) supported the hypothesis that lower levels of cholesterol are associated with major depressive disorders and suicidal behaviour.

Zhang, Muldoon, McKeown, and Cuffe (2005) showed that non-African American children between 6 and 16 years of age with low levels of cholesterol were almost three times more likely to have been suspended or expelled from schools than their peers with higher cholesterol levels The conclusion is that low total cholesterol may be a risk factor for aggression or a risk marker for other biologic variables that predispose to aggression.

The high refined carbohydrate diet plays havoc with the BSL. The BSL may not be necessarily too high, but rather too low, i.e. reactive hypoglycaemia. Carbohydrates produce a feeling of well-being and induce sleepiness. Sugar also can produce other effects such as:

- hyperactivity, anxiety, concentration difficulties, and crankiness in children,
- changes in brain waves, which can alter the mind's ability to think clearly, and
- depression.

Then there is the gluten, which is a protein found in grains. Many neurological illnesses are also associated with gluten.

Busby, Bold, Fellows, and Rostami (2018) showed that gluten is related to anxiety, depression, and other mood disorders, although this is mainly in those who have a gluten intolerance. In these individuals, a gluten free diet can help with their mood disorders.

There is another link between diet and these diseases. Refined, over processed foods, made from highly refined flour causes an overproduction of insulin as a response to the refined carbohydrate load. If there is also a gluten intolerance, this produces a double whammy. Sugar, and all ultra-processed dietary carbohydrates can cause hypoglycaemia if they form a major part of a meal. Since diet does cause metabolic derangements in children, which can produce behavioural issues, it is not hard to see that this will have a long-term effect on personality development.

Levitt Katz et al. (2005) showed that nearly one out of every five paediatric patients developing T2D also has a brain-development disorder, psychiatric illness, or behavioural disorder.

Dietary changes are needed.

Adults must take responsibility and remove sugar, grains, and dairy from children's diets. They must be encouraged to eat good, nutritious wholesome foods, not "junk food" such as pizza, fast food, and cola drinks (I refer to these as "black death!"). Should this happen, the children will develop more normally, have a clearer mind, their personality and behaviour will be better, and they will be less likely to develop into criminal, anti-social, aggressive people.

The sad thing is, that instead of correcting the diet, psychotropic medications are often prescribed. This treatment can only make the situation worse.

Statistics show that an increasing number of children and adolescents are taking drugs, not just illicit, but doctor prescribed medications. Many of these prescribed drugs are for mood disorders, notably depression, anxiety, autism, and ADD/ADHD. Teenagers are notoriously known to be moody and irritable. Do they really need drugs?

According to the British Office of National Statistics, prescriptions of psychiatric drugs have risen 400% since the mid-1990s. Data do indicate that during this same time, there was no corresponding increase in the incidence of mental illness among children.

The definition of depression is quite loose. Antidepressants do benefit some people but there are many on antidepressants who probably really do not need them; and there are some who react badly and suffer side effects, which can include homicidality and suicidality.

Are any of these drugs linked to violence?

Some antidepressants have been linked to hostility, aggression, homicide, homicidal thoughts, suicide, and suicidal thoughts. On October 15, 2004, the U.S. Food and Drug Administration (FDA) directed manufacturers of all antidepressant drugs to add "black box" warnings that describe the increased risk of suicide and suicidal thoughts in children and teens who take the drugs. Black box warnings are the most serious type placed on prescription medications.

The sad thing was that these drugs were prescribed for adolescents and children without any prior studies being conducted in these age groups.

There have been many violent massacres and

shootings, mostly in the USA. The Columbine School shooting, which is probably the best known, occurred on the 20th of April 1999. Twelve students and one teacher were killed, and 24 others were wounded. Antidepressant drugs have been implicated. One of the Columbine shooters, Eric Harris, was on some form of psychotropic medication.

This finding seems to be a common factor.

In the massacre at the Virginia Tech on 16 April 2007, the Chicago Tribune reports that Cho Seung Hui, who killed thirty-two fellow students, was taking antidepressant drugs.

In another shooting on 5 December 2007 in Omaha, the shooter, Robert Hawkins, had a history of being treated with psychiatric drugs for depression and ADHD.

Since then, there have been many mass shootings in the USA and most of these shooters were shown to have been either on or withdrawing from some form of psychotropic medications, specifically SSRIs.

The most common antidepressant drugs today are **S**elective **S**erotonin **R**euptake **I**nhibitors, or SSRIs. Serotonin is one of the brain's most important neurotransmitters and is thought to control everything from appetite to mood swings. The theory is that if you're depressed, compulsively eating or gambling, not sleeping properly or even just moody, you're probably lacking serotonin. It's important to note, however, that you can also have too much serotonin. The main role of SSRIs is to increase serotonin in the brain. However, some people react badly to SSRIs; in these instances, serotonin is raised too high and can act as an excitotoxin. When this happens, the excessive amount of serotonin produces side effects such as uncontrollable facial and body tics, dizziness, hallucinations, nausea, sexual dysfunction, addiction, electric-shock-like sensations in the brain and, of course, homicidal, or suicidal thoughts and behaviour.

These side effects were not emphasized. The drug manufacturers now warn that the drugs can cause homicidal ideation.

"We showed for the first time that SSRIs in comparison with placebo, increase aggression in children and adolescents, odds ratio 2.79 (95% CI 1.62 to 4.81). This is an important finding considering the many school shootings where the killers were on SSRIs" (Gøtzsche, 2017).

But then Hall et al. (2019) reports that there is no connection.

There are many articles on the internet divided between a connection or no connection.

Who do we believe?

The cynic in me says that certain big businesses do not want this information to be broadcast.

If in doubt ... don't

Unfortunately, many normal emotions are being diagnosed as a medical problem and are being medicated.

One SSRI (no names mentioned) has just entered *Australian Prescriber's* top 10 most prescribed medicines. More than 4.7 million prescriptions were issued between 2019 and 2020.

(https://www1.racgp.org.au/newsgp/clinical/an-antidepressant-is-now-one-of-australia-s-most- Accessed 06 September 2023)

Are so many people depressed, or do they just have

normal emotions that are being considered as a disease?

The word “depression” has been incorporated into the common vocabulary and is being overused, and probably misused.

Many of these people are not necessarily depressed: they may be “sad”, “unhappy”, “pessimistic”, “pissed off”, “feeling empty.” They go to their doctor and say they are “depressed”. Often ineffective, or no assessment is done before they are prescribed with an antidepressant medication: mainly because the modern doctor only knows pharmaceutical treatment.

These emotions need some sympathy, some understanding, some lifestyle changes, some omega 3 fatty acids, sunshine, and vitamin D: not necessarily drugs. Herbs such as St John’s Wort (*Hypericum perforatum*) may be used with mild to moderate symptoms (Apaydin et al., 2016).

When a person has symptoms that do not fit nicely into any physical illness, guess what? They are diagnosed with “depression” and treated with an antidepressant drug.

The current concept seems to be: if in doubt; give an antidepressant!

Autism

Autism is a neuro-developmental disorder that manifests itself before the age of three years. Children with autism are marked by impaired social interaction, impaired communication, and restricted and repetitive behaviour. They can stare into space for hours, throw tantrums, show no interest in people, and display repetitive purposeless actions such as hand flapping or head banging. They can be painfully sensitive to stimuli, including touch, taste, and sound, and frequently have little eye contact with others. They seem to live in a world by themselves.

The wide range of symptoms and severities reflects the complexity of the disorder, and it can be regarded as a spectrum disorder (autism spectrum disorders: ASD) which includes conditions such as Asperger's syndrome, Tourette's syndrome and Rett syndrome. Some are mild, some are severe. The cause(s) are not known but there are links to genetics, environment, especially Hg, diet and perhaps many more.

The numbers of autism diagnoses seem to be growing dramatically; however, we are not sure if the numbers are 1) actually growing, or 2) are we diagnosing it better or even 3) because the diagnosis criteria have changed to include larger numbers of children with any random abnormal behaviour.

The numbers are difficult to estimate. Estimates do vary from country to country and is complicated by varying criteria.

According to the Australian Bureau of Statistics (ABS) Survey of Disability, Ageing and Carers (SDAC), there is an overall prevalence rate of 0.7%, or about 1 in 150 people.

(https://www.aihw.gov.au › reports › disability › autism-in-australia › contents › autism - Accessed 18 Nov 2023)

As stated earlier, some cases of autism can be related to diet, especially gluten and casein (grains and dairy). There is also a controversial link to vaccines. Is it the vaccines causing minimal brain damage, or is it the thiomersal, a mercury-based preservative in vaccines? This preservative has now been removed.

What were they thinking when they decided to include a mercury-based preservative into vaccines designated for babies and children? Mercury (Hg) is the second most toxic element known.

Hg has been shown to cause brain damage.

The Australian government is encouraging the population to replace all incandescent light bulbs with the energy saving compact globes “to help protect the environment and reduce greenhouse gasses and global warming”. Their motives may be honourable but as usual they did not think it out fully. These globes are basically a mini fluorescent tube that can be fitted into standard light fittings. They do save power but there is a downside which is rarely discussed. These tubes are filled with a gas containing low-pressure Hg vapour and argon, or even krypton. The danger of these devices is the Hg, especially if one gets broken. What happens when they wear out? They get thrown into landfill and the Hg will escape and contaminate the groundwater. The rubbish dumps are now accepting these globes and are dealing with them separately.

In the USA, an estimated 600 million fluorescent lamps are disposed of annually into landfill amounting to 30,000 pounds of Hg waste. This amount is half the amount released into the atmosphere by coal-fired power plants each year! Again, what sounds like a good idea to save the planet from “global warming” can cause more toxic effects in the long run.

An interesting series of articles was written in the Washington Times (21 May 2005) about the fact that there is no, or very little, autism amongst the Amish population. The Amish are a religious group that keeps very much to themselves. They have religious exemption from mandatory vaccination.

There are about 22,000 Amish living in Lancaster County; and from the CDC figures of 1 in 166 rates of ASD, there should be over one hundred cases. The reporter only found a handful, and most of these had been vaccinated. Some others, who had not been vaccinated, were shown to have elevated levels of Hg in their bodies. Further investigations showed that they lived in the pathway of the smoke plume from a coal-fired power station that has been classed as one of the "dirtiest power plants" in the country. Hg is a by-product of coal combustion.

The Amish also isolate themselves from modern life. They do not drive cars, watch TV, or use phones. They do not eat store-bought meat: their meat is home grown without vaccines, growth hormones or antibiotics. Their vegetables are grown without chemicals or additives. They do take supplements.

They do spend time outside working, which leads to another interesting point.

Autism has been linked to vitamin D deficiency, which as we all know now, is due to avoidance of sun exposure.

Cannell (2017) wrote *"Children who are, or who are destined to become, autistic have lower 25(OH)D levels at 3 months of gestation, at birth and at age 8 compared to their unaffected siblings. Two open label trials found high dose vitamin D improves the core symptoms of autism in about 75% of autistic children."*

I am not advocating that we live exactly like the Amish, but we can learn from them. They eat clean foods, do not vaccinate, live a clean unpolluted life as much as possible, work, exercise, get plenty of sunshine, get enough sleep, have a great social community and support, and their health is good. If we can follow some of their lifestyle, then we can also benefit.

Sleep

All through this book I have been discussing the effect of sleep deprivation on health.

Lack of sleep is related to the development of MetS which, as we now know, manifests as obesity, diabetes, hypertension, and cancer. Though like many of the other things discussed in this book, it is the underlying metabolism that is the cause.

Lack of sleep can also cause behavioural problems in children and young adults. Youths who stay up late at night are more prone to anti-social behaviour, rule-breaking and attention problems (Susman et al., 2007; Hosokawa et al., 2022).

"Insomnia impairs cognitive and physical functioning and is associated with a wide range of impaired daytime functions across a number of emotional, social, and physical domains." (Roth, 2007).

Children need more sleep, but they are not getting it. There are too many distractions: they want to be up and watching TV or playing computer games. There is always an excuse. Some children say that they are just not tired. Is this perhaps because of a high sugar diet that has hyped them up? Just because adults stay up does not mean a child can; they do need more sleep.

In fact, adults as well need more sleep.

Babies and children are getting less sleep than they need, which makes them cranky and irritable the next day. Their brain is not as alert, and thinking may be cloudy. They will not function as well and, therefore, study and schooling can be affected. A child who has less sleep that they need can become hyper-excitable, less likely to listen or pay attention, and become emotionally erratic, very similar to the symptoms of ADD.

The epidemic of behavioural problems and mental health issues can be traced back to the abnormal conditions found in today's society. The diet, lifestyle, stress, and lack of sleep; all are a part of **Death by**

Civilization.

> *"Happiness is the highest form of health."*
> **Dalai Lama (1935-)**

> *"I have chosen to be happy because it is good for my health."*
> **Voltaire (1694-1778)**

TREATMENT

"The physician treats, but nature heals."
Hippocrates (c460 – c370 BCE)

All through this book, I have mentioned various things that you can do to help deal with, and to protect yourself and your family from these **diseases of civilization**. I have mentioned various minerals such as Cr, Mg, and Zn. I have mentioned vitamin C and vitamin D. I have made mention of various nutrients and herbs. This chapter is basically a summary of the different life-style changes, minerals, herbs, and vitamins that can be used to protect yourself from **Death by Civilization.**

Diet

The most important starting point is what we eat. Our species evolved/adapted to a certain eating pattern. Unfortunately, modern society has strayed away from this eating pattern and **diseases of civilization** have resulted. We need to get back to our hunter-gatherer roots and eat as close as possible as our ancestors did. This involves a higher protein, a higher fibre, a higher fat, and lower carbohydrate diet. The western style diet negatively affects the gut microbiome which can lead to/aggravate the development of MetS. Not only is the eating pattern what we eat but also what we should not eat. We should be grain free, sugar free and dairy free.

As mentioned before, there are those who eat grains and sugar, and drink milk without obvious adverse effects. It is possible that the onset of symptoms may be very subtle and may not be noticed. However, there are many who are not well and do not realise that their condition is related to their diet.

You may have noticed that all through this book I have been denigrating dairy. What I will say now is not to reverse that notion but to give a little bit of flexibility. Some people may want to drink some milk.

I can give some options.

Firstly, goat's and sheep's milk are a much better option than cow's milk.

The other option is A2 milk. This is cow's milk, but it comes from a distinct species of cow. A2 comes from the small Jersey or Guernsey cow, not from the big Friesian and Holstein cow.

In the past, many had a "house cow" in the backyard. Obviously, the smaller cow was better suited for a backyard than a big cow. It just so happens that these smaller cows make A2 milk. When the big corporations came onto the scene, they wanted a big cow, to make more milk to make more profit. The big cows make A1 milk. The difference between A1 and A2 is only 1 amino acid_(at position 67 there is a histidine instead of a proline) of the beta casein protein.

This one alteration does make a difference; it changes the shape the protein folds into, and shape is related to function. With this change in shape, when A1 is broken down, a peptide called *beta-casomorphine-7* (BCM-7) is created and this peptide has opioid properties. Opioids are known to have effects on the gut, e.g., constipation and on the brain, e.g., "brain fog". This can influence a proportion of the population. A1 milk consumption does cause increased gut issues in some, compared to A2 milk (Ho, Woodford, Kukuljan, & Pal, 2014).

Jianqin et al. (2016) wrote, *"Consumption of milk containing A1 β-casein was associated with increased gastrointestinal inflammation, worsening of PD3 (Post Dairy Digestive Discomfort) symptoms, delayed transit, and decreased cognitive processing speed and accuracy. Because elimination of A1 β-casein attenuated these effects, some symptoms of lactose intolerance may stem from inflammation it triggers and can be avoided by consuming milk containing only the A2 type of beta casein."*

The amino acid change in A1 milk is a mutation because humans, sheep, goat, and non-European cattle have the same protein structure of A2 milk.

A2 milk is less reactogenic than A1. I have seen this in practice: some children who are intolerant of normal milk can tolerate A2 better.

A2 milk is a better option if you want to drink milk.

I would suggest that you minimize milk consumption or do not drink it at all.

As soon as I say: *"Do not drink milk"* the first reaction is a panic; *"Where do I get my calcium from?"* This perception has been drummed into the general population and aided by the dairy corporation, more than likely to sell more milk, but how good a source of calcium (Ca) is milk?

This concern about Ca is largely because of the fear of osteoporosis. Again, the dairy corporation has advertised that milk drinking will protect from osteoporosis. How correct is this?

A study looked at the relation between dairy products and bone health in children. In 2005, Lanou, Berkow, and Barnard concluded that *"Scant evidence supports nutrition guidelines focused specifically on increasing milk or other dairy product intake for promoting child and adolescent bone mineralization."*

The 12-year Harvard Nurses' Health Study involving 78,000 nurses found that nurses who drank the most milk (two or more glasses per day) had a slightly higher risk of arm fracture (5% increase) and significantly higher risk of hip fracture (45% increase) (Feskanich, Willett, Stampfer, & Colditz, 1997).

So, we can see that the idea that you need dairy products for good bones is a myth.

This does not mean that Ca is not important. It is.

Non-dairy sources of Ca include:

- Nuts: almonds, macadamias, Brazil nuts, etc.,
- Vegetables, especially green leafy vegetables, broccoli, bok choy, wombok, etc.,
- Fish, especially with the bones: e.g., sardines,
- Bone broth.

Both Ca and phosphorus are needed for bone growth and strength, and it must be in the correct ratio of 2:1. The best source is bone itself, specifically the calcium/phosphorus crystal called *hydroxyapatite*. So, when you eat your sardines, or tuna or salmon … eat the bones as well! Another option is bone broth, which is relatively easy to make at home.

So, if you wish to supplement Ca, obtain a product that contains *"hydroxyapatite"*.

Of course, we must realise that vitamin D is essential for Ca and Mg absorption and utilisation.

The ideal diet should be meats, eggs, salads, vegetables, nuts, seeds, berries, fruits; all the foods our ancestors could hunt or gather.

> *Let food be thy medicine and medicine be thy food.*
> **Hippocrates (c460 – c370 BCE)**

Diets such as the original Banting diet (William Banting, 1796-1878), Atkin's diet, the protein power diet, the dinosaur gene diet, and even the CSIRO diet are largely based on the high(er) protein, low(er) carbohydrate diet.

There are some "foods" we should not be eating, or at least eat minimally. I have mentioned these many, many times but just so you don't forget, they are grains, dairy, and sugar.

Again, the best diet is not necessarily what we eat, but also what we *don't* eat.

The best source of our nutrients is our food. This would be so in a perfect world, but we do not live in a perfect world. The crops are grown in depleted soils, which means the produce is depleted in minerals. They then are picked green and ripen in the containers on the way to the shop. They are kept in cold storage for unknown lengths of time and are eventually placed on the shop shelves until they are bought only to sit in the fridge at home until eaten. How much nutrition is in the food? Probably much less than we think.

Another new problem with food is genetic modification (GM, genetically modified organisms, GMO). Officially GM foods have been certified by government agencies around the world to be safe. There are some activists, however, that maintain that we really do not know for sure. Many people distrust GMOs and denigrate them by calling them "Frankenfoods". Many people just do not trust the authorities. More years of research are needed, independent research. Research sponsored by big companies that produce these "foods" cannot always be trusted. Short term may be safe, but we do not know. Long term: we still are not sure.

If in doubt ... don't.

Do not mess around with nature. In the film *"I am Legend"* a genetically modified virus is developed as a cure for cancer. The virus gets out of hand and kills off most of the human race! The remaining population turn into zombie-like creatures. Could this happen in real life?

Unfortunately, we may not even know if we are eating GM foods because the corporations are fighting tooth and nail to have GM products unlabelled.

Is this so people cannot choose and actively boycott these products? Would *you* buy the product if it is labelled as GMO?

The best form of food is GM free, fresh, organic (pesticide and chemical free) produce.

Organic is better.

Studies have confirmed what we suspected.

"Consequently, it can be concluded that organically produced plant derived food products have a higher nutritional value, including antioxidants than conventional ones. Furthermore, due to the fact that there is a lower level of contamination in organic crops, the risk of diseases caused by contaminated food is significantly reduced" (Györéné, Varga, & Lugasi, 2006).

"On average, organic food of plant origin is characterized by a trace presence of pesticides, a lower content of nitrates and an increased content of polyphenols and vitamin C. Organic products of animal origin contain more beneficial for health unsaturated fatty acid" (Glibowski, 2020).

"Comparing the analyses of tomatoes from conventional and organic production systems demonstrated statistically higher levels ($P < 0.05$) of phenolic compounds in organic tomatoes" (Vallverdú-Queralt, Jáuregui, Medina-Remón, & Lamuela-Raventós, 2012).

Another aspect of eating is *not* eating, that is - fasting.

Horne et al. (2018) showed that fasting reduced the

incidence of coronary artery disease and diabetes. This study looked at Mormons who fast for 24 hours on the first Sunday of the month. Of course, Mormons do not drink or smoke either (though these factors were considered), and the fasting makes an increased difference, which all adds up to the fact that Mormons are less likely to die of heart disease than the average American.

This makes sense. Our ancestors did not have a regular dietary intake, there were times where there was nothing to eat at all, i.e. a non-voluntary fast. Not eating for a short time is a part of our physiology. We are generally eating too much, too often, now, as compared to our ancestors. Missing out a meal now and then can be beneficial. This eating pattern is referred to as "intermittent fasting". Not eating for a time will reduce the insulin levels, this will give our pancreas a "rest" and this is a possible reason why fasting can reduce heart disease.

Studies looking at Muslims during the fasting month of Ramadan showed positive benefits on the markers of cardiovascular disease (Jahrami et al., 2021; Aksungar, Eren, Ure, Teskin, & Ates, 2005; Saleh et al., 2004).

As I said earlier, the diet is not just what we eat but also what we shouldn't eat but now we can see that occasionally it is beneficial not to eat at all!

> *"Instead of using medicine, better fast today."*
> **Plutarch (c46 – after 119 CE)**

Even though we should be getting all our nutrients from our food, for the reasons already discussed, supplements and herbs may still be a good idea. I will discuss some of the more important ones.

Chromium (Cr)

To the average person, Cr is the stuff car bumper bars were made from! It is a trace element and its importance in human health was discovered by accident. During the early days of total parenteral nutrition (TPN), where patients were totally nourished on an intravenous feeding solution, it was discovered that some patients developed high blood sugars. The elevated blood sugars persisted despite the giving of insulin. The role of Cr was known from animal research, so Cr was added to the TPN solution. The elevated blood sugars went down to normal. Cr was elevated to the status of an essential nutrient for humans.

I should point out here that I am not referring to hexavalent Cr, which is carcinogenic, but to trivalent Cr which is the essential nutrient.

The exact mode of action of Cr is not known for sure, but its action is on the insulin receptor. Receptors are sites on the cell surface where hormones can attach. They are specific sites like a lock and key and once the hormone attaches to its specific site, the action of the hormone can be carried out. Cr does not work by stimulating the production of more insulin. It works on insulin already present, making its action more efficient by encouraging the insulin receptor to start working again.

As we know, the underlying defect in MetS is IR: the insulin receptor has switched off. Cr can help switch the receptor back on, therefore, Cr supplementation can assist in all the symptoms of MetS.

"Chromium is an essential nutrient involved in the metabolism of glucose, insulin and blood lipids. Suboptimal dietary intake of chromium is associated with increased risk factors associated with diabetes and cardiovascular diseases." "Chromium increases insulin binding to cells, insulin receptor number and activates insulin receptor kinase leading to increased insulin sensitivity" (Anderson, 2000).

"Several studies have now demonstrated that chromium supplements enhance the metabolic action of insulin and lower some of the risk factors for cardiovascular disease, particularly in overweight individuals. Chromium picolinate, specifically, has been shown to reduce insulin resistance and to help reduce the risk of cardiovascular disease and type 2 diabetes" (Havel, 2004).

Cr is sparse in the western diet, the best sources being organ meats, mushrooms, wheat germ, broccoli, and processed meats. It is important to point out that these sources, especially the plant sources, are dependent on the soil content of Cr. No Cr in the soil, therefore no Cr in the broccoli!

Our paleolithic ancestors probably ate more Cr in their diet because they ate the organs as well as the meat of the animals they hunted, which very few do today and the vegetables they ate were not grown in depleted soils.

Another factor to be considered is that today much of the Cr is lost in the urine. The ingestion of sugars and the rise in insulin levels cause Cr to be excreted in the urine and we do eat more sugar than we ought! We become Cr deficient.

Not only are we ingesting less Cr, but we are also excreting more. No wonder we have low levels of this trace mineral, and no wonder that we have an epidemic of diabetes, obesity, heart disease, and cancer.

Magnesium (Mg)

Magnesium (Mg) deficiency is a well-known phenomenon in diabetes: it is especially prominent in those with poor control of the diabetes, as well as complications, such as retinopathy, neuropathy, and cardiac disease.

Mg is lost in excess amounts in the urine,

- due to glycosuria (high amount of glucose in the urine). This works in much the same way as diuretics: high urinary output and the loss of many minerals. (In fact, diuretics can also produce Mg loss.) and
- hyperinsulinaemia itself influences reducing Mg levels. Insulin resistant cells are resistant to the Mg entering the cell and since Mg is an intra cellular mineral, if it cannot get into the cell then it is urinated out.

This is an especially important mineral. It is a cofactor in over three hundred enzyme reactions, it improves insulin sensitivity (conversely, a lack of Mg is related to IR) and insulin secretion but there is controversy about its action on diabetic control.

Sales, Pedrosa, Lima, Lemos, and Colli (2011) demonstrated that supplementing Mg plays a significant role in blood sugar control.

Rodríguez-Morán and Guerrero-Romero (2003) showed that those who were supplemented with 50 mls of magnesium chloride solution (50 grams Mg per 1,000mls solution, which is equivalent to 2,500 mg of Mg daily!!!) showed improvement in serum Mg levels, glycaemic control and HbA1c levels.

Many of the studies are not consistent. Perhaps the problem is that not all diabetics are Mg deficient to the same degree. Only about 25-38% of those with T2D are hypomagnesic, these are the ones more likely to develop complications. These are the ones that need higher doses, used for longer periods, to prevent complications, and improve control (de Lordes Lina et al., 1998).

Sales and Pedrosa (2006) showed that Mg has a substantial role in diabetes prevention, as well as, preventing, or reducing, some of the complications of diabetes. Low levels of Mg may play a role in the development of retinopathy, hypertension, nephropathy, stroke and altered platelet function.

As Mg is an intracellular mineral, measuring serum levels are useless. When ordering a Mg level, a red blood cell (RBC) Mg should be requested, not a serum Mg. Mg levels can be monitored, and appropriate doses given.

Zinc (Zn)

Zinc (Zn) is also another important mineral. It is a cofactor in over two hundred enzyme reactions and is involved in virtually all aspects of insulin metabolism, synthesis, secretion, and utilisation. As with Mg, Zn levels are also lower in diabetics. Diabetics tend to have low Zn levels largely due to increased Zn excretion in the urine. Zn deficiency is related to IR and has a bearing on immunity. Zn improves lymphocyte function which has a role in immunity and infection prevention.

Zn is also needed in collagen formation, therefore is a factor in normal healing.

I should highlight the fact that diabetics tend to have poor immunity and to heal poorly.

From this we see that Zn is lost in diabetics, but the important question is: *"Does Zn supplementation improve the situation?"* It is logical to think that since Zn is needed for diabetic function and Zn is low in diabetics, then replacing the Zn will make it all better.

Not necessarily so!

Giving large doses of Zn can make the situation worse. Raz, Karsai, and Katz (1989) supplemented Zn as zinc sulphate, 220 mg 3 times a day (this is equivalent to 149 mg of elemental Zn daily, which is a huge dose) to T2D patients. In the end diabetic control was worse.

In another study, Cunningham, Fu, Mearkle, and Brown (1994) supplemented Zn at 50 mg elemental Zn daily. After 28 days the HbA1c was higher, meaning a worsening of the diabetic state.

However, when a more normal dose of Zn (30 mg) was supplemented, there was a decrease in parameters of oxidative stress, though no change in diabetic control. The Zn may not necessarily improve diabetic control but does improve oxidative stress which may help in preventing long term complications (Roussel et al., 2003).

Many of the complications of diabetes are caused by intracellular oxidation and free radical damage caused by Zn deficiency and loss of Zn dependent antioxidant enzymes. Zn supplementation may protect against the complications but not necessarily alter the diabetic state itself.

Zn needs to be supplemented, not just for diabetics but everyone. A recommended dose of 15-30 mg of elemental Zn is needed daily.

As we have seen above, diabetics are a special category: it seems that in diabetics, we shouldn't supplement more than 30 mg per day as it could worsen the situation.

Vanadium (V)

Vanadium (V) is a trace mineral that has been shown to have an insulin mimic action and is related to molybdenum and tungsten which also have similar actions.

V has also been shown to improve the body's sensitivity to insulin in both type 1 and 2 diabetics and to lower cholesterol and blood pressure. The problem is that the research is still uncertain about dosage. V is thought to act as a *phosphatase* inhibitor which affects kinases which are *"critical to other hormones that also act on common parts of the insulin pathway"* (Treviño & Diaz, 2020).

See also Thompson et al., 2009; Treviño et al., 2019.

Selenium (Se)

Selenium (Se) is a trace mineral that is essential for good health. Se is a cofactor in various enzymes, especially glutathione peroxidase, which acts as an antioxidant that helps prevent cellular damage. Se is found in various foods, especially Brazil nuts, garlic, meat, fish, and eggs. However, note that the level of Se in meat or in plants depends entirely on the level of Se in the soil. There are parts of the world which have adequate Se in the soil. Those that live there do not need Se supplementation.

Australia and New Zealand are very Se deficient and, therefore, most people need to take a Se supplement. An intake below 400 μg/day is considered safe for almost all individuals. Se can be toxic in high doses, so supplementation must be carefully supervised (See, Lavercombe, Dillon, & Ginsberg, 2006).

Earlier studies on Se showed that supplementation reduced the incidence of cancer, most likely because of its antioxidant effects.

In a study of Se supplementation and skin cancer, the researchers found no benefit in preventing skin cancer but found significant protection for cancers at other sites (lung, colorectal and prostate) and *"significant reduction in total cancer mortality"* (Clark et al., 1996).

Newer studies show that it may not be useful. Vinceti et al. (2018) concludes *"Overall, there is no evidence to suggest that increasing selenium intake through diet or supplementation prevents cancer in humans. However, more research is needed to assess whether selenium may modify the risk of cancer in individuals with a specific genetic background or nutritional status, and to investigate possible differential effects of various forms of selenium."*

However, an even newer study shows that Se may be helpful. Kuria et al. (2020) concluded that *"The findings in this study suggest that selenium is protective against cancer however the effects vary with different cancers."*

Panchal, Wanyonyi, and Brown (2017) discuss the use of Se, V, and Cr *"that may play crucial roles in controlling blood glucose concentrations possibly through their insulin-mimetic effects."*

Vitamin C

Vitamin C is another important nutrient that I have discussed before. It is an extremely important nutrient, and it should be looked at as a nutrient, not as a vitamin.

Calling it a vitamin gives the impression that it is needed in small doses but really it is a nutrient and needed in larger doses. Vitamin C has antioxidant properties, which help protect the body from free-radical damage.

Vitamin C has been shown to help correct IR and endothelial dysfunction in cardiac and diabetic patients.

Also, it can protect against the long-term damage caused by MetS.

Damage is caused by oxidative stress. Vitamin C, in conjunction with other antioxidants, can protect the body against free radical damage.

"Oxidative stress may play a role in the pathophysiology of diabetes and cardiovascular disease, but little is known about antioxidant status among individuals with the metabolic syndrome who are at high risk for developing these conditions."

"After adjusting for age, sex, race or ethnicity, education, smoking status, cotinine concentration, physical activity, fruit and vegetable intake, and vitamin or mineral use, participants with the metabolic syndrome had significantly lower concentrations of retinyl esters, vitamin C, and carotenoids, except lycopene. With additional adjustment for serum lipid concentrations, vitamin E concentrations were

significantly lower in participants with the metabolic syndrome than those without the syndrome. Retinol concentrations were similar between the two groups. After excluding participants with diabetes, the results were very similar. Consumption of fruits and vegetables was also lower among people with the metabolic syndrome. Adults with the metabolic syndrome have suboptimal concentrations of several antioxidants, which may partially explain their increased risk for diabetes and cardiovascular disease" (Ford, Mokdad, Giles, & Brown, 2003).

High dose intravenous vitamin C has been shown to improve symptoms and prolong life in patients with terminal cancer (Casciari et al., 2001).

Padayattyu et al. (2006) published three case histories of terminal cancer patients treated with intravenous vitamin C.

"In light of recent clinical pharmacokinetic findings and in vitro evidence of anti-tumour mechanisms, these case reports indicate that the role of high-dose intravenous vitamin C therapy in cancer treatment should be reassessed."

Vitamin D

I have discussed vitamin D quite extensively in the book. The major source is from the action of sunlight onto the skin. Unfortunately, people are sun-paranoid, and a large percentage of the population is vitamin D deficient.

Vitamin D does have a relationship with heart disease, diabetes, and cancer.

"This paper highlights the relationship of vitamin D insufficiency with cardiovascular disease and non-insulin dependent diabetes mellitus, two diseases that account for up to 50% of all deaths in western countries" (Zittermann, 2006).

"Vitamin D and calcium insufficiency may negatively influence glycemia, whereas combined supplementation with both nutrients may be beneficial in optimizing glucose metabolism" (Pittas, Lau, Hu, & Dawson-Hughes, 2007).

Fish oil/omega 3 fatty acids

Fish oils exert important biological effects on the body, in normal people, as well as in diabetics. Fish oil has a beneficial action on the cell membranes, and this in turn has a positive effect on the cell receptors, that is, it can help to prevent diabetes and it helps the insulin receptor to recover. It also is beneficial in preventing some of the complications of diabetes and/or MetS: heart disease, strokes, peripheral neuropathy and vasculopathy.

Unfortunately, the western diet is too high in omega 6 fatty acids. This is largely due to the plant oils and grains in the diet. Our ancestors lived on a diet where the omega 3 to omega 6 ratio was about 1:1, the western diet is now 1:40 or even higher. We are eating the wrong oils. We need to eat more omega 3 and less omega 6.

"Excessive amounts of omega 6 PUFA (poly unsaturated fatty acid) and a very high omega6/omega 3 ratio, as is found in today's Western diets, promote the pathogenesis of many diseases, including cardiovascular disease, cancer, and inflammatory and autoimmune disease, whereas increased levels of omega 3 PUFA (a low omega 6/omega 3 ratio) exert suppressive effects" (Simopoulos, 2002).

Omega 6 comes from grains, cereals, plant oils (corn, sunflower, safflower, canola), whole grain products, baked goods, and margarine. Unfortunately, we are told that they are healthy, and we are even encouraged to consume them because they are "cholesterol free".

This is based mainly on commercial interests. Fair to say that omega 6 is not bad in itself, but the amount is the problem. The omega 3/omega 6 ratio is what is important.

Many of the commercially produced meats are grain fed. Chickens are fed on chicken pellets, mostly based on grains, which have a high omega 6 content, therefore the meat is also high in omega 6, and so are the eggs.

Our ancestors hunted animals that were free range. Therefore, the animals ate their natural diet and their meat, and eggs were high in omega 3. So, if you want to eat healthy, eat free range meats, deep sea fish (wild caught and not farmed), kangaroo (because it is culled not farmed, therefore free range), and lamb (young, grass fed, not feed lotted). Free range chooks scratch and forage, eating bugs and grubs and plants, the natural diet of chooks. These chooks have a higher amount of omega 3 in their meat and so do their eggs.

Yam, Eliraz, and Berry (1996) concluded that *"Israel has one of the highest dietary polyunsaturated/saturated fat ratios in the world; the consumption of omega-6 polyunsaturated fatty acids (PUFA) is about 8% higher than in the USA, and 10-12% higher than in most European countries. In fact, Israeli Jews may be regarded as <u>a population-based dietary experiment of the effect of a high omega-6 PUFA diet</u>, a diet that until recently was widely recommended."* (emphasis the author)

The researchers go on to say that there is a high incidence in the Israeli population of cardiovascular disease, hypertension, T2D, and obesity, which are all associated with IR and hyperinsulinaemia, which is MetS. There is also an increased incidence of cancer especially in women.

There is some evidence that omega 3 fatty acids can decrease IR.

Let's correct our omega 3 to omega 6 ratio, eat more omega 3 and less omega 6. We can see that these oils do influence the progress of MetS. Fish oil can be supplemented or even better, eat more fish, especially sardines.

N acetyl Cysteine (NAC)

N acetyl cysteine (NAC) is a sulphur containing amino acid and is the precursor of glutathione, the body's main detoxifier. NAC also has activity against oxidative stress and inflammation. There is also a beneficial activity for brain function, especially glutamate dysfunction.

NAC has been shown to be beneficial for addiction and substance abuse, schizophrenia, obsessive-compulsive disorders (OCD) and mood disorders, including depression and anxiety.

Ooi, Green, and Pak (2018) discuss that oxidative stress and reduced antioxidant status is common to many psychiatric disorders, including schizophrenia, depression, bipolar and OCD.

Glutathione is the body's most important detoxifier especially in the liver but can also have an action on the brain. NAC as a precursor to glutathione can be considered as a "brain detoxifier". Any brain, psychiatric issues can be related to brain dysfunction. NAC can reduce inflammation and has antioxidant activity as well as modulating the glutamatergic system, which has been linked to many psychiatric disorders.

NAC (800-2400 mg daily) showed improvement in autism. "*... suggest increased social behavior, decreased aggression, and decreased self-harm, facilitating lowering of doses of antipsychotics in males with ASD aged 4–17 years*" (Bradlow, Berk, Kalivas, Back, & Kanaan, 2022).

NAC is also used in paracetamol (acetaminophen) and with death cap mushroom (Amanita phalloides) poisoning as a liver protectant. NAC is also useful in chronic respiratory conditions such as chronic obstructive pulmonary disease, idiopathic pulmonary fibrosis, bronchiectasis, chronic bronchitis, and cystic fibrosis, as a mucolytic agent.

As mental health issues are becoming more common, NAC may be a useful nutrient in treating these conditions. Safe doses range from 600 mg to 2,800 mg depending on age and condition.

Tryptophan

Tryptophan is an essential amino acid that is the precursor of serotonin and melatonin. Tryptophan is converted to 5 hydroxytryptophan (5 HTP). This is achieved by the enzyme *tryptophan hydroxylase.* This enzyme needs cofactors iron (Fe), Ca, vitamin B3 and 5 methyltetrahydrofolate (5 MTHF), 5 HTP is converted to serotonin by *dopa decarboxylase*, which has cofactors Zn, Mg, vitamin B6 and vitamin C. Serotonin to melatonin is a more complex reaction, but the cofactors are s adenosylmethionine (SAMe), and vitamin B5.

As you can see there are some common nutrients needed for these reactions, Zn, Mg, B complex, SAMe, and 5 MTHF. Note that 5 MTHF is the only form of folate the body can use. The folate in the diet is converted to 5 MTHF, though not everyone can do this efficiently due to a genetic variation of the MTHFR gene.

One of the issues with tryptophan is that it can go down three pathways, so supplementing vitamin B3 can encourage the reaction to go down the serotonin pathway.

Alternatively, a related supplement can be used: 5HTP.

An interesting note is that in mainstream psychiatry, in cases which respond poorly to SSRIs, 5 MTHF is being used as adjunct therapy (Papakostas et al., 2012). Another nutrient that mainstream psychiatry is using in resistant cases of depression is SAMe (Papakostas, Mischoulon, Shyu, Alpert, & Fava, 2010).

I hope you can see the rationale for the use of these nutrients.

Doses – tryptophan 500 mg to 1,000 mg. Using too much tryptophan may cause unwanted effects, as the large dose of tryptophan can be forced to go down the kynurenine pathway because t*ryptophan hydroxylase* is the rate limiting step in the tryptophan to 5 HTP reaction.

5 HTP doses are much smaller; 100 - 200 mg daily.

Medicinal cannabis (MC)

Medicinal cannabis (MC) usage has been increasing rapidly over the last few years. After being banned for many years, cannabis is now being considered for medicinal purposes. Cannabis has many components: there are hundreds of cannabinoids, terpenes, flavonoids which all work together known as the "entourage effect". The two main cannabinoids are cannabidiol (CBD) and tetrahydrocannabinol (THC). THC has a psychoactive effect and that is probably the main reason it was banned many years ago. CBD has many properties: it has anti-inflammatory, analgesic, anti-anxiety, and relaxing effects and it does not have a psychoactive action. All through this book I have discussed that inflammation is a part of MetS. I have discussed various substances that can be used for its anti-inflammatory effect such as curcumin, fish oil and ashwagandha. CBD can be added to that list.

Wiciński et al. (2023) writes that although some studies are contradictory, there is adequate evidence that CBD can have positive effects on treating many aspects of MetS, including blood pressure, diabetes, cholesterol, obesity, and fatty liver. An important factor is that CBD has been shown to be very safe. CBD does not only have effects on the cannabis receptors, but interacts with many other receptors, thus producing its wide-ranging effects. CBD has been described as being very promiscuous because of its ability to interact with many receptors.

St Mary's thistle

St Mary's thistle *(Silybum marianum)* also known as milk thistle, Marian's thistle, holy thistle, and blessed thistle, has been used for liver problems for an extremely long time, going as far back as the ancient Greeks and Romans. Modern research has confirmed what these ancient healers knew; that is that this herb is extremely useful for liver problems.

This herb can help in healing most liver problems, anything from the serious, such as cirrhosis, viral hepatitis, alcoholic hepatitis, and fatty liver, to the minor and anything in-between. Extracts of this herb have been shown to protect the liver from one of the most hepatotoxic of substances, the death cap mushroom.

St Mary's thistle works in three ways:

- Powerful antioxidants (silymarin and silybin, the "active ingredients") in the herb prevent liver damage by preventing free radical damage,
- increases the levels of glutathione in the liver, which is especially important for

detoxification of many toxic substances and,
- stimulates the re-generation of new liver cells.

New research has also shown that St Mary's thistle influences diabetes and glycaemic control. This makes sense because the liver participates in sugar metabolism. The liver is possibly one of the first organs that becomes insulin resistant: this herb helps to prevent this and help achieve normal metabolism. Hueseini et al. (2006) showed that St Mary's thistle did improve glycaemic control in type 2 diabetics.

Gymnema sylvestre

Gymnema sylvestre (also known as gurmar: Hindi for "destroyer of sugar") is an ayurvedic herb that has been used for centuries to treat sugar problems. New research has confirmed what the ancient healers knew: this herb does influence sugar. How it works is not yet fully determined but research has shown that the herb works on many levels.

- Increases insulin stimulation by the pancreas. Animal studies have shown that this may be due to regeneration of the pancreatic beta cells.

- Increases the activity of enzymes involved with glucose absorption, so it possibly may influence the insulin receptor.
- Can help to repair liver function.
- Reduces intestinal sugar absorption.
- Chewing the leaves of the plant affects the taste buds which blocks sweetness craving, as well as reducing appetite generally.

In one study, diabetics taking glucose-lowering drugs were also given Gymnema leaf extracts. All the patients benefited from significant reductions in glucose and glycosylated haemoglobin after taking Gymnema for 18 months. In fact, 5 of the patients were able to safely discontinue taking their glucose-reducing drugs as long as they kept taking Gymnema. The subjects reported that they were more alert, less exhausted and had an overall better sense of well-being (Baskaran, Kizar Ahamath, Radha Shanmugasundaram, & Shanmugasundaram, 1990).

Momordica charanta

Momordica charanta, also known as the bitter melon, has been shown to be useful in the treatment of diabetes. The vine grows in Asia, India, Africa, and the Caribbean and has been used in these cultures for a very long time both as a part of traditional cooking and as a medicine. Studies of this fruit have shown it to be useful in the treatment of diabetes, though most of the studies have been non-randomised and non-controlled.

"Bitter gourd (Momordica charantia) is a vegetable with pantropical distribution. It contains substances with antidiabetic properties such as charantin, vicine, and polypeptide-p, as well as other unspecific bioactive components such as antioxidants. Metabolic and hypoglycemic effects of bitter gourd extracts have been demonstrated in cell culture, animal, and human studies. The mechanism of action, whether it is via regulation of insulin release or altered glucose metabolism and its insulin-like effect, is still under debate" (Krawinkel & Keding, 2006).

"The effect of karela (Momordica charantia), a fruit indigenous to South America and Asia, on glucose and insulin concentrations was studied in nine non-insulin-dependent diabetics and six non-diabetic laboratory rats. A water-soluble extract of the fruits significantly reduced blood glucose concentrations

during a 50gm oral glucose tolerance test in the diabetics and after force-feeding in the rats. Fried karela fruits consumed as a daily supplement to the diet produced a small but significant improvement in glucose tolerance. Improvement in glucose tolerance was not associated with an increase in serum insulin responses. These results show that karela improves glucose tolerance in diabetes. Doctors supervising Asian diabetics should be aware of the fruit's hypoglycaemic properties" (Leatherdale et al., 1981).

"Investigations were carried out to evaluate the effect of Momordica charantia on the glucose tolerance of maturity onset diabetic patients. The fruit juice of M. charantia was found to significantly improve the glucose tolerance of 73% of the patients investigated while the other 27% failed to respond" (Welihinda, Karunanayake, Sheriff, & Jayasinghe, 1986).

Cinnamon

Cinnamon (*Cinnamomum aromaticum),* a spice that is in virtually every one's kitchen cupboard, has a significant effect on sugar levels (Kirkham, Akilen, Sharma, & Tsiami, 2009).

"The results of this study demonstrate that intake

of 1, 3, or 6 g of cinnamon per day reduces serum glucose, triglyceride, LDL cholesterol, and total cholesterol in people with type 2 diabetes and suggest that the inclusion of cinnamon in the diet of people with type 2 diabetes will reduce risk factors associated with diabetes and cardiovascular diseases" (Khan, Safdar, Ali Khan, Khattak, & Anderson, 2003).

A hydroxychalcone derived from cinnamon seems to increase insulin receptor sensitivity (Jarvill-Taylor, Anderson, & Graves, 2001).

As the underlying problem with MetS is IR, cinnamon not only helps diabetes, but can improve IR in general.

The use of this spice is very easy; just add small amounts into your cooking, into your coffee, tea, etc.

The addition of cinnamon will only add to the benefits of diet, and the vitamins and minerals and herbs you are taking.

Cinnamon, however, does highlight one of the issues with herbs. Not everyone can take it. In Chinese terminology, cinnamon is a *yang* herb: very heating. To give this herb to a *yang* person, i.e. a hot, sweaty type person will only increase the heat and increase discomfort. Cinnamon is suited to a *yin* person; a cold type and the herb will heat them up.

Ashwagandha

Ashwagandha has been used for thousands of years in the Ayurvedic system of medicine in India. This herb may not specifically deal with MetS but as an adaptogen, helps the body deal with stress, which is rife in today's society. All through the book I have been discussing how stress can have negative effects on the body. Treating stress can be a very helpful part of treating MetS. Ashwagandha does not remove the stress but helps the body cope better with it. It can increase energy and can help to promote sleep. Ashwagandha also has anti-inflammatory properties.

Of course, we should not forget more sunshine, more exercise, more sleep, and less stress.

CONCLUSION

We have become a very unhealthy species. Chronic health problems, such as diabetes, obesity, heart disease and cancer are rife. Diseases that in the past only affected the elderly are now developing in younger and younger populations.

Death rates are growing from **diseases of civilization**.

Our ability to reproduce is being compromised: a portion of the population has already become infertile: this is shown by the increase in the need for fertility clinics and in-vitro fertilization. Another portion of the population can still reproduce but the progeny is increasingly becoming unhealthier.

The overall health of the population is very poor. This is leading to our possible extinction.

Our brains, our minds, which for a long time have been our greatest asset, to achieve all the things we have done, are now failing. We were so smart to use chemistry and physics and science to make all these technological wonders but, unfortunately, we weren't smart enough to look to the future and appreciate the negative consequences of our actions.

Our minds are suffering from the side effects of the diet, the pollution, the lack of sleep and the stress. Mental illness is rife and growing. How can a society survive if a large proportion of the population is mentally affected?

The sad thing is that this is caused by something as fundamental as our diet and our lifestyle. Our species evolved as hunter-gatherers, who adapted to a unique lifestyle. A diet which is higher in protein and fat and lower in carbohydrates, a very active lifestyle, in less continuously stressful surroundings, who could sleep more and lived in a much cleaner environment.

What is happening now?

We are being encouraged to eat a diet totally foreign to our physiology and to our digestive systems. The mismatch between what we should be eating and what we are eating is causing a large part of the problem.

We are becoming lazier … and why not? There are so many labour-saving devices being invented. Exercise was a particularly important part of our ancestral lifestyle. This significant decrease in exercise is contributing to **Death by Civilization**.

We live in an incredibly stressful and polluted world.

Genetics change very slowly; we are genetically still paleolithic people. We have not yet adapted to this modern world, and it is this modern world that is killing us.

The question is: will we evolve fast enough to be able to cope with these changes before we die out? Will we evolve or adapt fast enough to be able to cope with all the dietary changes, stress, and pollution that we ourselves have unleashed?

There have been fantastic technological changes, which on one hand is a boon for us, while on the other hand, it is leading to our demise. The pollution, the release of heavy metals, the invention and manufacture of totally new chemicals that have permeated the whole eco-sphere, has brought some benefit, although perhaps only in the short-term because we are now paying the price. We are now realizing the ecological damage these compounds can do to our environment and to us.

Who wins? In the short term, some become very rich.

In the long term, no one wins.

In the end, we all, rich and poor, become victims of **Death by Civilization.**

The population keeps growing but the health of our nation is deteriorating. Chronic disease is increasing, and most of this chronic disease is related to our diet, our lifestyle and to the pollution that is produced by the technological world we live in.

We can make some changes; but these would interfere with the profits of the great powerful multinational corporations.

Anything healthy is against profits.

The changes we need to make are to look after our diet, improve our lifestyle and minimize our exposure to pollution.

After reading this book, hopefully you will have the knowledge not only to know what to do but also why you should do it.

SUMMARY

Eat better

Fast occasionally

Exercise more

Sleep more

Stress out less

Avoid pollution

Sunshine exposure not sunburn

Supplement vitamins and minerals

Herbs are safer than pharmaceuticals

REFERENCES

Adan, R., van der Beek, E., Buitelaar, J., Cryan, J., Hebebrand, J., Higgs, S., … Dickson, S. (2019). Nutritional psychiatry: Towards improving mental health by what you eat. *Eur Neuropsychopharmacol, 29*(12), 1321-1332. doi: 10.1016/j.euroneuro.2019.10.011

Aksungar, F., Eren, A., Ure, S., Teskin, O. & Ates, G. (2005). Effects of intermittent fasting on serum lipid levels, coagulation status and plasma homocysteine levels. *Ann Nutr Metab, 49*(2), 77-82. doi: 10.1159/000084739

Al-Khudairy, L., Flowers, N., Wheelhouse, R., Ghannam, O., Hartley, L., Stranges, S., Rees, K. (2017). Vitamin C supplementation for the primary prevention of cardiovascular disease. *Cochrane Database Syst Rev, 3*(3), CD011114. doi: 10.1002/14651858.CD011114.pub2

Almgren, T., Persson, B., Wilhelmsen, L., Rosengren,

A. & Andersson, O. (2005). Stroke and coronary heart disease in treated hypertension -- a prospective cohort study over three decades. *J Intern Med, 257*(6), 496-502. doi: 10.1111/j.1365-2796.2005.01497.x

Alp, H., Soner, B., Baysal, T. & Şahin, A. (2015). Protective effects of Hawthorn (Crataegus oxyacantha) extract against digoxin-induced arrhythmias in rats. *Anatol J Cardiol, 15*(12), 970-5. doi: 10.5152/akd.2014.5869

Anderson, R. (2000). Chromium in the prevention and control of diabetes. *Diabetes Metab, 26*(1), 22-7

Andersson, O., Almgren, T., Persson, B., Samuelsson, O., Hedner, T. & Wilhelmsen, L. (1998). Survival in treated hypertension: follow up study after two decades. *BMJ, 317*(7152), 167-71. doi: 10.1136/bmj.317.7152.167

Angelidi, A., Belanger, M., Kokkinos, A., Koliaki, C. & Mantzoros, C. (2022) Novel noninvasive approaches to the treatment of obesity: From pharmacotherapy to gene therapy. *Endocr Rev, 43*(3), 507-557. doi: 10.1210/endrev/bnab034

Ansari, F., Pourjafar, H., Tabrizi, A. & Homayouni, A. (2020). The effects of probiotics and prebiotics on mental disorders: A review on depression, anxiety, Alzheimer, and autism spectrum disorders. *Curr Pharm*

Biotechnol, 21(7), 555-565. doi: 10.2174/1389201021666200107113812

Apaydin, E., Maher, A., Shanman, R., Booth, M., Miles, J., Sorbero, M. & Hempel, S. (2016). A systematic review of St. John's wort for major depressive disorder. *Syst Rev, 5*(1), 148. doi: 10.1186/s13643-016-0325-2

Arab, A. & Mostafalou, S. (2023). Pesticides and insulin resistance-related metabolic diseases: Evidences and mechanisms. *Pestic Biochem Physiol, 195*, 105521. doi: 10.1016/j.pestbp.2023.105521

Avgerinos, K., Spyrou, N., Mantzoros, C. & Dalamaga, M. (2019). Obesity and cancer risk: Emerging biological mechanisms and perspectives. *Metabolism, 92*, 121-135. doi: 10.1016/j.metabol.2018.11.001

Ayas, N., White, D., Al-Delaimy, W., Manson, J., Stampfer, M., Speizer, F., … Hu, F. (2003). A prospective study of self-reported sleep duration and incident diabetes in women. *Diabetes Care, 26*(2), 380-4. doi: 10.2337/diacare.26.2.380

Balachandar, R., Pullakhandam, R., Kulkarni, B. & Sachdev, H. (2021). Relative efficacy of vitamin D_2 and vitamin D_3 in improving vitamin D status: Systematic review and meta-analysis. *Nutrients,*

13(10), 3328. doi: 10.3390/nu13103328

Balwierz, R., Biernat, P., Jasińska-Balwierz, A., Siodłak, D., Kusakiewicz-Dawid, A., Kurek-Górecka, A., … Ochędzan-Siodłak, W. (2023). Potential Carcinogens in Makeup Cosmetics. *Int J Environ Res Public Health, 20*(6), 4780. doi: 10.3390/ijerph20064780

Banks, W., Coon, A., Robinson, S., Moinuddin, A., Shultz JM, Nakaoke, R. & Morley, J. (2004). Triglycerides induce leptin resistance at the blood-brain barrier. *Diabetes, 53*(5), 1253-60. doi: 10.2337/diabetes.53.5.1253

Baskaran, K., Kizar Ahamath, B., Radha Shanmugasundaram, K. & Shanmugasundaram, E. (1990). Antidiabetic effect of a leaf extract from Gymnema sylvestre in non-insulin-dependent diabetes mellitus patients. *J Ethnopharmacol, 30*(3), 295-300. doi: 10.1016/0378-8741(90)90108-6

Bataille, V., Boniol, M., De Vries, E., Severi, G., Brandberg, Y., … Autier, P. (2005). A multicentre epidemiological study on sunbed use and cutaneous melanoma in Europe. *Eur J Cancer, 41*(14), 2141-9. doi: 10.1016/j.ejca.2005.04.038

Bateman, B., Warner, J., Hutchinson, E., Dean, T.,

Rowlandson, P., Gant, C., … Stevenson, J. (2004). The effects of a double blind, placebo controlled, artificial food colourings and benzoate preservative challenge on hyperactivity in a general population sample of preschool children. *Arch Dis Child, 89*(6), 506-11. doi: 10.1136/adc.2003.031435

Beckett, N., Nunes, M. & Bulpitt, C. (2000). Is it advantageous to lower cholesterol in the elderly hypertensive? *Cardiovasc Drugs Ther, 14*(4), 397-405. doi: 10.1023/a:1007812232328

Beckley, A., Caspi, A., Broadbent, J., Harrington, H., Houts, R., Poulton, R., … Moffitt, T. (2018). Association of childhood blood lead levels with criminal offending. *JAMA Pediatr, 172*(2), 166-173. doi: 10.1001/jamapediatrics.2017.4005

Bellastella, G., Scappaticcio, L., Esposito, K., Giugliano, D. & Maiorino, M. (2018). Metabolic syndrome and cancer: "The common soil hypothesis". *Diabetes Res Clin Pract, 143*, 389-397. doi: 10.1016/j.diabres.2018.05.024

Beral, V.; Million Women Study Collaborators. (2003). Breast cancer and hormone-replacement therapy in the Million Women Study. *Lancet, 362*(9382), 419-27. doi: 10.1016/s0140-6736(03)14065-2

Beresford, S., Weiss, N., Voigt, L. & McKnight, B. (1997). Risk of endometrial cancer in relation to use of oestrogen combined with cyclic progestagen therapy in postmenopausal women. *Lancet, 349*(9050), 458-61. doi: 10.1016/S0140-6736(96)07365-5

Berrino, F., Bellati, C., Secreto, G., Camerini, E., Pala, V., Panico, S., … Kaaks, R. (2001). Reducing bioavailable sex hormones through a comprehensive change in diet: the diet and androgens (DIANA) randomized trial. *Cancer Epidemiol Biomarkers Prev, 10*(1), 25-33.

Berwick, M., Armstrong, B., Ben-Porat, L., Fine, J., Kricker, A., Eberle, C, & Barnhill, R. (2005). Sun exposure and mortality from melanoma. *J Natl Cancer Inst, 97*(3), 195-9. doi: 10.1093/jnci/dji019

Billups, K., Bank, A., Padma-Nathan, H., Katz, S. & Williams, R. (2005). Erectile dysfunction is a marker for cardiovascular disease: results of the minority health institute expert advisory panel. *J Sex Med, 2*(1), 40-50; discussion 50-2. doi: 10.1111/j.1743-6109.2005.20104_1.x

Black, R., Spence, M., McMahon, R., Cuskelly, G., Ennis, C., McCance, D., … Hunter, S. (2006). Effect of eucaloric high- and low-sucrose diets with identical macronutrient profile on insulin resistance and vascular risk: a randomized controlled trial. *Diabetes, 55*(12), 3566-72. doi: 10.2337/db06-0220

Blackburn, H. (2021). John 'Jack' Gofman. Researcher and Social Activist.: 'Fair-haired Boy' and 'Enemy Within'. *Am J Cardiol, S0002-9149*(21)00531-2. doi: 10.1016/j.amjcard.2021.05.051

Blatt, J., Van Le, L., Weiner, T. & Sailer, S. (2003). Ovarian carcinoma in an adolescent with transgenerational exposure to diethylstilbestrol. *J Pediatr Hematol Oncol, 25*(8), 635-6. doi: 10.1097/00043426-200308000-00009

Blot, W., Li, J., Taylor, P., Guo, W., Dawsey, S., Wang, G., … Li, G. (1993). Nutrition intervention trials in Linxian, China: supplementation with specific vitamin/mineral combinations, cancer incidence, and disease-specific mortality in the general population. *J Natl Cancer Inst, 85*(18), 1483-92. doi: 10.1093/jnci/85.18.1483

Boney, C., Verma, A., Tucker, R. & Vohr, B. (2005). Metabolic syndrome in childhood: association with birth weight, maternal obesity, and gestational diabetes mellitus. *Pediatrics, 115*(3), e290-6. doi: 10.1542/peds.2004-1808

Bradlow, R., Berk, M., Kalivas, P., Back, S. & Kanaan,

R. (2022). The Potential of N-Acetyl-L-Cysteine (NAC) in the Treatment of Psychiatric Disorders. *CNS Drugs, 36*(5), 451-482. doi: 10.1007/s40263-022-00907-3

Breakey, J. (1997). The role of diet and behaviour in childhood. *J Paediatr Child Health, 33*(3), 190-4. doi: 10.1111/j.1440-1754.1997.tb01578.x

Broom, G., Shaw, I. & Rucklidge, J. (2019). The ketogenic diet as a potential treatment and prevention strategy for Alzheimer's disease. *Nutrition, 60*, 118-121. doi: 10.1016/j.nut.2018.10.003

Broughton, D. & Moley, K. (2017). Obesity and female infertility: potential mediators of obesity's impact. *Fertil Steril, 107*(4), 840-847. doi: 10.1016/j.fertnstert.2017.01.017

Brouns, F. & Shewry, P. (2022). Do gluten peptides stimulate weight gain in humans? *Nutr Bull, 47*(2), 186-198. doi: 10.1111/nbu.12558

Bruckert, E., Giral, P., Heshmati, H. & Turpin, G. (1996). Men treated with hypolipidaemic drugs complain more frequently of erectile dysfunction. *J Clin Pharm Ther, 21*(2), 89-94. doi: 10.1111/j.1365-2710.1996.tb00006.x

Bruckert, E., Giral, P., Heshmati, H. & Turpin, G.

(1996). Men treated with hypolipidaemic drugs complain more frequently of erectile dysfunction. *J Clin Pharm Ther, 21*(2), 89-94. doi: 10.1111/j.1365-2710.1996.tb00006.x

Bungau, A., Radu, A., Bungau, S., Vesa, C., Tit, D. & Endres, L. (2023). Oxidative stress and metabolic syndrome in acne vulgaris: Pathogenetic connections and potential role of dietary supplements and phytochemicals. *Biomed Pharmacother, 164*, 115003. doi: 10.1016/j.biopha.2023.115003

Bungau, S., Tit, D., Vesa, C., Abid, A., Szilagyi, D., Radu, A., … Endres L. (2022). Non-conventional therapeutical approaches to acne vulgaris related to its association with metabolic disorders. *Eur J Pharmacol, 923*, 174936. doi: 10.1016/j.ejphar.2022.174936

Burstin, F. & Allison, L. (2006). Now it's not enough sun. *Adelaide Advertiser*, 26 April, 8.

Busby, E., Bold, J., Fellows, L. & Rostami, K. (2018). Mood disorders and gluten: It's not all in your mind! A systematic review with meta-analysis. *Nutrients, 10*(11), 1708. doi: 10.3390/nu10111708

Byard, R. (2012). The complex spectrum of forensic issues arising from obesity. *Forensic Sci Med Pathol, 8*(4), 402-13. doi: 10.1007/s12024-012-9322-5

Byrne, P., Demasi, M., Jones, M., Smith, S., O'Brien, K. & DuBroff, R. (2022). Evaluating the association between low-density lipoprotein cholesterol reduction and relative and absolute effects of statin treatment: A systematic review and meta-analysis. *JAMA Intern Med, 182*(5), 474-481. doi: 10.1001/jamainternmed.2022.0134

Bytyçi, I., Penson, P., Mikhailidis, D., Wong, N., Hernandez, A., Sahebkar, A., … Banach M. (2022). Prevalence of statin intolerance: a meta-analysis. *Eur Heart J, 43*(34), 3213-3223. doi: 10.1093/eurheartj/ehac015

Caballero, A. (2003). Endothelial dysfunction in obesity and insulin resistance: a road to diabetes and heart disease. *Obes Res, 11*(11), 1278-89. doi: 10.1038/oby.2003.174

Cabrera, S., Mindell, J., Toledo, M., Alvo, M. & Ferro, C. (2016). Associations of blood pressure with geographical latitude, solar radiation, and ambient temperature: Results from the Chilean health survey, 2009-2010. *Am J Epidemiol, 183*(11), 1071-3. doi: 10.1093/aje/kww037

Cai, X., Wang, C., Yu, W., Fan, W., Wang, S., Shen, N., … Wang, F. (2016). Selenium exposure and cancer risk: An updated meta-analysis and meta-regression.

Sci Rep, 6, 19213. doi: 10.1038/srep19213

Cannell, J. (2017). Vitamin D and autism, what's new? *Rev Endocr Metab Disord, 18*(2), 183-193. doi: 10.1007/s11154-017-9409-0

Carrara, D., Bruno, R., Bacca, A., Taddei, S., Duranti, E., Ghiadoni, L. & Bernini, G. (2016). Cholecalciferol treatment downregulates renin-angiotensin system and improves endothelial function in essential hypertensive patients with hypovitaminosid D. *J Hypertens, 34*(11), 2199-205. doi: 10.1097/HJH.0000000000001072

Carrera-Lanestosa, A., Moguel-Ordóñez, Y. & Segura-Campos, M. (2017). Stevia rebaudiana Bertoni: A natural alternative for treating diseases associated with metabolic syndrome. *J Med Food, 20*(10), 933-943. doi: 10.1089/jmf.2016.0171

Casciari, J., Riordan, N., Schmidt, T., Meng, X., Jackson, J. & Riordan, H. (2001). Cytotoxicity of ascorbate, lipoic acid, and other antioxidants in hollow fibre in vitro tumours. *Br J Cancer, 84*(11), 1544-50. doi: 10.1054/bjoc.2001.1814

Castelli, W. (1992). Concerning the possibility of a nut. *Arch Intern Med, 152*(7), 1371-2.

Cech, I., Holguin, A., Sokolow, H. & Smith, V. (1984). Selenium availability in Texas: possible clinical significance. *South Med J, 77*(11), 1415-20. doi: 10.1097/00007611-198411000-00016

Cederberg, H., Stančáková, A., Yaluri, N., Modi, S., Kuusisto, J. & Laakso, M. (2015). Increased risk of diabetes with statin treatment is associated with impaired insulin sensitivity and insulin secretion: a 6 year follow-up study of the METSIM cohort. *Diabetologia, 58*(5), 1109-17. doi: 10.1007/s00125-015-3528-5

Cersosimo, E. & DeFronzo, R. (2006). Insulin resistance and endothelial dysfunction: the road map to cardiovascular diseases. *Diabetes Metab Res Rev, 22*(6), 423-36. doi: 10.1002/dmrr.634

Champagne, C. (2008). Magnesium in hypertension, cardiovascular disease, metabolic syndrome, and other conditions: a review. *Nutr Clin Pract, 23*(2), 142-51. doi: 10.1177/0884533608314533

Chandola, T., Brunner, E. & Marmot, M. (2006). Chronic stress at work and the metabolic syndrome: prospective study. *BMJ, 332*(7540), 521-5. doi: 10.1136/bmj.38693.435301.80

Chang, C., Benson, M. & Fam, M. (2017). A review of Agent Orange and its associated oncologic risk of genitourinary cancers. *Urol Oncol, 35*(11), 633-639. doi: 10.1016/j.urolonc.2017.08.029

Chang, C., Ho, S., Chiu, H. & Yang, C. (2011). Statins increase the risk of prostate cancer: a population-based case-control study. *Prostate, 71*(16), 1818-24. doi: 10.1002/pros.21401

Che, T., Yan, C., Tian, D., Zhang, X., Liu, X. & Wu, Z. (2012). The association between sleep and metabolic syndrome: A systematic review and meta-analysis. *Front Endocrinol (Lausanne), 12*, 773646. doi: 10.3389/fendo.2021.773646

Chen, L., Qiao, Q., Zhang, S., Chen, Y., Chao, G. & Fang, L. (2012). Metabolic syndrome and gallstone disease. *World J Gastroenterol, 18*(31), 4215-20. doi: 10.3748/wjg.v18.i31.4215

Chen, Q., Lin, R., Hong, X., Ye, L. & Lin, Q. (2016). Treatment and prevention of inflammatory responses and oxidative stress in patients with obstructive sleep apnea hypopnea syndrome using Chinese herbal medicines. *Exp Ther Med, 12*(3), 1572-1578. doi: 10.3892/etm.2016.3484

Cheraghi, Z., Doosti-Irani, A., Almasi-Hashiani, A., Baigi, V., Mansournia, N., Etminan, M. & Mansournia, M. (2019). The effect of alcohol on osteoporosis: A systematic review and meta-analysis. *Drug Alcohol Depend, 197*, 197-202. doi: 10.1016/j.drugalcdep.2019.01.025

Chiu, K., Chu, A., Go, V. & Saad, M. (2004). Hypovitaminosis D is associated with insulin resistance and beta cell dysfunction. *Am J Clin Nutr, 79*(5), 820-5. doi: 10.1093/ajcn/79.5.820

Choi, Y., Moskowitz, J., Myung, S., Lee, Y. & Hong, Y. (2020). Cellular phone use and risk of tumors: Systematic review and meta-Analysis. *Int J Environ Res Public Health, 17*(21), 8079. doi: 10.3390/ijerph17218079

Church, T. (2011). Exercise in obesity, metabolic syndrome, and diabetes. *Prog Cardiovasc Dis, 53*(6), 412-8. doi: 10.1016/j.pcad.2011.03.013

Ciok, J. & Dolna, A. (2006). Znaczenie indeksu glikemicznego w ocenie gospodarki weglowodanowej [The role of glycemic index concept in carbohydrate metabolism]. *Przegl Lek, 63*(5), 287-91. Polish.

Clark, L., Combs, G. Jr., Turnbull, B., Slate, E., Chalker, D., Chow, J., … Taylor, J. (1996). Effects of selenium supplementation for cancer prevention in patients with carcinoma of the skin. A randomized controlled trial. Nutritional Prevention of Cancer Study Group. *JAMA, 276*(24), 1957-63

Cloud, A., Vilcins, D. & McEwen, B. (2020). The effect of hawthorn (Crataegus spp) on blood pressure: A systemic review. *Adv Integ Med, 7*(3), 167-175. doi:

10.1016/j.aimed.2019.09.002

Cohn, J., Kamili, A., Wat, E., Chung, R. & Tandy, S. (2010). Dietary phospholipids and intestinal cholesterol absorption. *Nutrients, 2*(2), 116-27. doi: 10.3390/nu2020116

Conforti, C., Agozzino, M., Emendato, G., Fai, A., Fichera, F., Marangi, G., … Dianzani, C. (2022). Acne and diet: a review. *Int J Dermatol, 61*(8), 930-934. doi: 10.1111/ijd.15862

Cordain, L., Eades, M. & Eades, M. (2003). Hyperinsulinemic diseases of civilization: more than just syndrome X. *Comp Biochem Physiol A Mol Integr Physiol, 136*(1), 95-112. doi: 10.1016/s1095-6433(03)00011-4

Cordain, L., Eaton, S., Sebastian, A., Mann, N., Lindeberg, S., Watkins, B., … Brand-Miller, J. (2005). Origins and evolution of the Western diet: health implications for the 21st century. *Am J Clin Nutr, 81*(2), 341-54. doi: 10.1093/ajcn.81.2.341

Cormick, G., Ciapponi, A., Cafferata, M., Cormick, M. & Belizán, J. (2022). Calcium supplementation for prevention of primary hypertension. *Cochrane Database Syst Rev, 1*(1), CD010037. doi: 10.1002/14651858.CD010037.pub4

Correia, A. & Vale, N. (2022). Tryptophan Metabolism in Depression: A Narrative Review with a Focus on Serotonin and Kynurenine Pathways. *Int J Mol Sci, 23*(15), 8493. doi: 10.3390/ijms23158493

Cox, F., Misiou, A., Vierkant, A., Ale-Agha, N., Grandoch, M., Haendeler, J. & Altschmied, J. (2020). Protective effects of curcumin in cardiovascular diseases-impact on oxidative stress and mitochondria. *Cells, 11*(3), 342. doi: 10.3390/cells11030342

Craft, S. (2005). Insulin resistance syndrome and Alzheimer's disease: age- and obesity-related effects on memory, amyloid, and inflammation. *Neurobiol Aging, 26* Suppl 1, 65-9. doi: 10.1016/j.neurobiolaging.2005.08.021

Crichton, G., Alkerwi, A. & Elias, M. (2015). Diet soft drink consumption is associated with the metabolic syndrome: A two sample comparison. *Nutrients, 7*(5), 3569-86. doi: 10.3390/nu7053569

Cruz, A., Amatuzio, D., Grande, F., & Hay, L. (1961). Effect of intra-arterial insulin on tissue cholesterol and fatty acids in alloxan-diabetic dogs. *Circ Res, 9*, 39-43. doi: 10.1161/01.res.9.1.39

Culver, A., Ockene, I., Balasubramanian, R., Olendzki, B., Sepavich, D., Wactawski-Wende, J., … Ma, Y. (2012). Statin use and risk of diabetes mellitus in postmenopausal women in the Women's Health Initiative. *Arch Intern Med, 172*(2),144-52. doi: 10.1001/archinternmed.2011.625

Cunningham, J., Fu, A., Mearkle, P. & Brown, R. (1994). Hyperzincuria in individuals with insulin-dependent diabetes mellitus: concurrent zinc status and the effect of high-dose zinc supplementation. *Metabolism, 43*(12), 1558-62. doi: 10.1016/0026-0495(94)90016-7

Dabke K, Hendrick G, Devkota S. The gut microbiome and metabolic syndrome. *J Clin Invest, 129*(10), 4050-4057. doi: 10.1172/JCI129194

Dai S, Mo Y, Wang Y, Xiang B, Liao Q, Zhou M, … Zeng Z. (2020). Chronic stress promotes cancer development. *Front Oncol, 10*, 1492. doi: 10.3389/fonc.2020.01492

Dandona, P., Chaudhuri, A., Mohanty, P. & Ghanim, H. (2007). Anti-inflammatory effects of insulin. *Curr Opin Clin Nutr Metab Care, 10*(4), 511-7. doi: 10.1097/MCO.0b013e3281e38774

Dandona, P., Aljada, A, & Bandyopadhyay, A. (2004). Inflammation: the link between insulin resistance, obesity and diabetes. *Trends Immunol, 25*(1), 4-7. doi: 10.1016/j.it.2003.10.013

Das, G., Crocombe, S., McGrath, M., Berry, J. & Mughal, M. (2006). Hypovitaminosis D among healthy adolescent girls attending an inner city school. *Arch Dis Child, 91*(7), 569-72. doi: 10.1136/adc.2005.077974

Davis, R., Rogers, M., Coates, A., Leung, G. & Bonham, M. (2022). The impact of meal timing on risk of weight gain and development of obesity: a review of the current evidence and opportunities for dietary intervention. *Curr Diab Rep, 22*(4), 147-155. doi: 10.1007/s11892-022-01457-0

Debras, C., Chazelas, E., Srour, B., Druesne-Pecollo, N., Esseddik, Y., Szabo de Edelenyi, F., … Touvier, M. (2022). Artificial sweeteners and cancer risk: Results from the NutriNet-Santé population-based cohort study. *PLoS Med, 19*(3), e1003950. doi: 10.1371/journal.pmed.1003950

Debras, C., Chazelas, E., Srour, B., Kesse-Guyot, E., Julia, C., Zelek, L., … Touvier, M. (2020). Total and added sugar intakes, sugar types, and cancer risk: results from the prospective NutriNet-Santé cohort. *Am J Clin Nutr, 112*(5), 1267-1279. doi: 10.1093/ajcn/nqaa246

de la Rubia Ortí, J., García-Pardo, M., Drehmer, E., Sancho Cantus, D., Julián Rochina, M., Aguilar, M. & Hu Yang, I. (2018). Improvement of main cognitive functions in patients with Alzheimer's disease after treatment with coconut oil enriched Mediterranean diet: A pilot study. *J Alzheimers Dis, 65*(2), 577-587. doi: 10.3233/JAD-180184

de la Rubia Ortí, J., Sánchez Álvarez, C., Selvi Sabater, P., Bueno Cayo, A., Sancho Castillo, S., Rochina, M. & Hu Yang, I. (2017). Influencia del aceite de coco en enfermos de alzhéimer a nivel cognitivo [How does coconut oil affect cognitive performance in alzheimer patients?]. *Nutr Hosp, 34*(2), 352-356. Spanish. doi: 10.20960/nh.780

De Giorgi, R., Rizzo Pesci, N., Quinton, A., De Crescenzo, F., Cowen, P. & Harmer, C. (2021). Statins in depression: An evidence-based overview of mechanisms and clinical studies. *Front Psychiatry, 12*, 702617. doi: 10.3389/fpsyt.2021.702617

de Graaf, L., Brouwers, A. & Diemont, W. (2004). Is decreased libido associated with the use of HMG-CoA-reductase inhibitors? *Br J Clin Pharmacol, 58*(3), 326-8. doi: 10.1111/j.1365-2125.2004.02128.x

De Long, N. & Holloway, A. (2017). Early-life chemical exposures and risk of metabolic syndrome. *Diabetes Metab Syndr Obes, 10*, 101-109. doi: 10.2147/DMSO.S95296 de Lordes Lima, M., Cruz, T., Pousada, J., Rodrigues, L., Barbosa, K. & Canguçu, V. (1998). The effect of magnesium supplementation in increasing doses on the control of type 2 diabetes. *Diabetes Care, 21*(5), 682-6. doi: 10.2337/diacare.21.5.682

de Lorgeril, M., Salen, P., Caillat-Vallet, E., Hanauer, M., Barthelemy, JC. & Mamelle, N. (1997). Control of bias in dietary trial to prevent coronary recurrences: The Lyon Diet Heart Study. *Eur J Clin Nutr, 51*(2), 116-22. doi: 10.1038/sj.ejcn.1600374

de Lorgeril, M., Salen, P., Martin, J., Monjaud, I., Boucher, P. & Mamelle, N. (1998). Mediterranean dietary pattern in a randomized trial: prolonged survival and possible reduced cancer rate. *Arch Intern Med, 158*(11), 1181-7. doi: 10.1001/archinte.158.11.1181

de Lorgeril, M., Salen, P., Martin, J., Monjaud, I., Delaye, J. & Mamelle, N. (1999). Mediterranean diet, traditional risk factors, and the rate of cardiovascular complications after myocardial infarction: final report of the Lyon Diet Heart Study. *Circulation, 99*(6), 779-85. doi: 10.1161/01.cir.99.6.779

DiNicolantonio, J. & O'Keefe, J. (2022). Added sugars drive insulin resistance, hyperinsulinemia, hypertension, type 2 diabetes and coronary heart disease. *Mo Med, 119*(6), 519-523.

Desoto, M. & Hitlan, R. (2007). Blood levels of mercury are related to diagnosis of autism: a reanalysis of an important data set. *J Child Neurol, 22*(11), 1308-11. doi: 10.1177/0883073807307111

D'Eufemia, P., Celli, M., Finocchiaro, R., Pacifico, L., Viozzi, L., Zaccagnini, M., … Giardini O. (1996). Abnormal intestinal permeability in children with autism. *Acta Paediatr, 85*(9), 1076-9. doi: 10.1111/j.1651-2227.1996.tb14220.x

Diamond, D. & Leaverton, P. (2023). Historical review of the use of relative risk statistics in the portrayal of the purported hazards of high LDL cholesterol and the benefits of lipid-lowering therapy. *Cureus, 15*(5), e38391. doi: 10.7759/cureus.38391

Diamond, J. (1987). The Worst Mistake in the History of the Human Race. *Discover Magazine,* May, 64-66.

Dibaba, D., Xun, P., Song, Y., Rosanoff, A., Shechter, M. & He, K. (2017). The effect of magnesium supplementation on blood pressure in individuals with insulin resistance, prediabetes, or noncommunicable chronic diseases: a meta-analysis of randomized controlled trials. *Am J Clin Nutr, 106*(3), 921-929. doi: 10.3945/ajcn.117.155291

DiNicolantonio, J, Lucan, S. & O'Keefe, J. (2016). The

evidence for saturated fat and for sugar related to coronary heart disease. *Prog Cardiovasc Dis, 58*(5), 464-72. doi: 10.1016/j.pcad.2015.11.006

DiNicolantonio, J., Mehta, V., Zaman, S. & O'Keefe, J. (2018). Not salt but sugar as aetiological in osteoporosis: A review. *Mo Med, 115*(3), 247-252.

Doherty, E. (2007). High risk as mums get bigger. *Adelaide Sunday Mail,* 14 Jan, 22.

Dong, S., Wang, Z., Shen, K. & Chen, X. (2021). Metabolic syndrome and breast cancer: Prevalence, treatment response, and prognosis. *Front Oncol, 11*, 629666. doi: 10.3389/fonc.2021.629666

Doody, M., Lonstein, J., Stovall, M., Hacker, D., Luckyanov, N. & Land, C. (2000). Breast cancer mortality after diagnostic radiography: findings from the U.S. Scoliosis Cohort Study. *Spine (Phila Pa 1976), 25*(16), 2052-63. doi: 10.1097/00007632-200008150-00009

Draper, G., Vincent, T., Kroll, M. & Swanson, J. (2005). Childhood cancer in relation to distance from high voltage power lines in England and Wales: a case-control study. *BMJ, 330*(7503), 1290. doi: 10.1136/bmj.330.7503.1290

Drewnowski, A. & Darmon, N. (2005). Food choices

and diet costs: an economic analysis. *J Nutr, 135*(4), 900-4. doi: 10.1093/jn/135.4.900

Drewnowski, A. & Specter, S. (2004). Poverty and obesity: the role of energy density and energy costs. *Am J Clin Nutr, 79*(1), 6-16. doi: 10.1093/ajcn/79.1.6

DuBroff, R., Malhotra, A. & de Lorgeril, M. (Hit or miss: the new cholesterol targets. BMJ Evid Based Med. 2021 Dec;26(6):271-278. doi: 10.1136/bmjebm-2020-111413

Eddy, D., Schlessinger, L., Kahn, R., Peskin, B. & Schiebinger, R. (2009). Relationship of insulin resistance and related metabolic variables to coronary artery disease: a mathematical analysis. *Diabetes Care, 32*(2), 361-6. doi: 10.2337/dc08-0854

Ellis, P. (2019). The story of gallstones and their treatment. *J Perioper Pract, 29*(11), 382-384. doi: 10.1177/1750458919838450

Ellison, L., & Morrison, H. (2001). Low serum cholesterol concentration and risk of suicide. *Epidemiology, 12*(2), 168-72. doi: 10.1097/00001648-200103000-00007

Engelberg, H. (1992). Low serum cholesterol and suicide. *Lancet, 339*(8795), 727-9. doi: 10.1016/0140-6736(92)90609-7

Eskenazi, B., Gunier, R., Rauch, S., Kogut, K., Perito, E., Mendez, X., … Mora, A. (2023). Association of lifetime exposure to glyphosate and aminomethylphosphonic acid (AMPA) with liver inflammation and metabolic syndrome at young adulthood: Findings from the CHAMACOS study. *Environ Health Perspect, 131*(3), 37001. doi: 10.1289/EHP11721

Esposito, K. & Giugliano, D. (2004). The metabolic syndrome and inflammation: association or causation? *Nutr Metab Cardiovasc Dis, 14*(5), 228-32. doi: 10.1016/s0939-4753(04)80048-6

Extramiana, F. & Leenhardt, A. (2022). Fish oil and risk of atrial fibrillation: yet another paragon of the association or causation dilemma. *Eur J Prev Cardiol, zwac243*. doi: 10.1093/eurjpc/zwac243

Ezkurdia, A., Ramírez, M. & Solas, M. (2023). Metabolic syndrome as a risk factor for Alzheimer's disease: A focus on insulin resistance. *Int J Mol Sci, 24*(5), 4354. doi: 10.3390/ijms24054354

Fatehi Hassanabad, A. (2019). Current perspectives on statins as potential anti-cancer therapeutics: clinical outcomes and underlying molecular mechanisms. *Transl Lung Cancer Res, 8*(5), 692-699. doi: 10.21037/tlcr.2019.09.08

Fernando, G., Martha, R. & Evangelina, R. (1999). Consumption of soft drinks with phosphoric acid as a risk factor for the development of hypocalcemia in postmenopausal women. *J Clin Epidemiol, 52*(10), 1007-10. doi: 10.1016/s0895-4356(99)00097-9

Fernando, W., Martins, I., Goozee, K., Brennan, C., Jayasena, V. & Martins, R. (2015). The role of dietary coconut for the prevention and treatment of Alzheimer's disease: potential mechanisms of action. *Br J Nutr, 114*(1), 1-14. doi: 10.1017/S0007114515001452

Feskanich, D., Willett, W., Stampfer, M. & Colditz, G. (1997). Milk, dietary calcium, and bone fractures in women: a 12-year prospective study. *Am J Public Health, 87*(6), 992-7. doi: 10.2105/ajph.87.6.992

Feychting, M., Osterlund, B. & Ahlbom, A. (1998). Reduced cancer incidence among the blind. *Epidemiology, 9*(5), 490-4.

Filipski, E., King, V., Li, X., Granda, T., Mormont, M., Liu, X., … Lévi, F. (2002). Host circadian clock as a control point in tumor progression. *J Natl Cancer Inst, 94*(9), 690-7. doi: 10.1093/jnci/94.9.690

Fishel, M., Watson, G., Montine, T., Wang, Q., Green, P., Kulstad, J., … Craft S. (2005). Hyperinsulinemia provokes synchronous increases in central inflammation and beta-amyloid in normal adults. *Arch Neurol, 62*(10), 1539-44. doi: 10.1001/archneur.62.10.noc50112

Folkers, K., Langsjoen, P., Willis, R., Richardson, P., Xia, L., Ye, C., & Tamagawa, H. (1990). Lovastatin decreases coenzyme Q levels in humans. *Proc Natl Acad Sci U S A, 87*(22), 8931-4. doi: 10.1073/pnas.87.22.8931

Ford, E., Mokdad, A., Giles, W. & Brown, D. (2003). The metabolic syndrome and antioxidant concentrations: findings from the Third National Health and Nutrition Examination Survey. *Diabetes, 52*(9), 2346-52. doi: 10.2337/diabetes.52.9.2346

Fournier, A., Berrino, F. & Clavel-Chapelon, F. (2008). Unequal risks for breast cancer associated with different hormone replacement therapies: results from the E3N cohort study. *Breast Cancer Res Treat, 107*(1), 103-11. doi: 10.1007/s10549-007-9523-x

Fox, C., Meigs, J., D'Agostino, R., Gaziano, J.& Vasan R. (2007) Soft drink consumption and risk of developing cardiometabolic risk factors and the metabolic syndrome in middle-aged adults in the community. *Circulation, 116*(5), 480-8. doi: 10.1161/CIRCULATIONAHA.107.689935

Fox, C., Pencina, M., Meigs, J., Vasan, R., Levitzky, Y.

& D'Agostino, R. Sr. (2006). Trends in the incidence of type 2 diabetes mellitus from the 1970s to the 1990s: the Framingham Heart Study. *Circulation, 113*(25), 2914-8. doi: 10.1161/CIRCULATIONAHA.106.613828

Framnes, S. & Arble, D. (2018). The bidirectional relationship between obstructive sleep apnoea and metabolic disease. *Front Endocrinol (Lausanne), 9*, 440. doi: 10.3389/fendo.2018.00440

Franceschi, S., Favero, A., La Vecchia, C., Negri, E., Conti, E., Montella, M., … Decarli, A. (1997). Food groups and risk of colorectal cancer in Italy. *Int J Cancer, 72*(1), 56-61. doi: 10.1002/(sici)1097-0215(19970703)72:1<56::aid-ijc8>3.0.co;2-3

Franceschi, S., Favero, A., Parpinel, M., Giacosa, A. & La Vecchia, C. (1998). Italian study on colorectal cancer with emphasis on influence of cereals. *Eur J Cancer Prev, 7* Suppl 2, S19-23. doi: 10.1097/00008469-199805000-00004

Fraser, G., Jacobsen, B., Knutsen, S., Mashchak, A. & Lloren, J. (2020). Tomato consumption and intake of lycopene as predictors of the incidence of prostate cancer: the Adventist Health Study-2. *Cancer Causes Control, 31*(4), 341-351. doi: 10.1007/s10552-020-01279-z

Freedland, S., Grubb, K., You, S., Humphreys, E., Nielsen, M., Mangold, L., … Partin, A. (2005). Obesity and risk of biochemical progression following radical prostatectomy at a tertiary care referral center. *J Urol, 174*(3), 919-22. doi: 10.1097/01.ju.0000169459.78982.d7

Freire, R., Fernandes, L., Silva, R., Coelho, B., de Araújo. L., Ribeiro, L., … Alvarez-Leite, J. (2016). Wheat gluten intake increases weight gain and adiposity associated with reduced thermogenesis and energy expenditure in an animal model of obesity. *Int J Obes (Lond), 40*(3), 479-86. doi: 10.1038/ijo.2015.204

Gaines, J., Vgontzas, A., Fernandez-Mendoza, J., He, F., Calhoun, S., Liao, D. & Bixler, E. (2017). Increased inflammation from childhood to adolescence predicts sleep apnea in boys: A preliminary study. *Brain Behav Immun, 64*, 259-265. doi: 10.1016/j.bbi.2017.04.011

Gala, T. & Seaman, D. (2011). Lifestyle modifications and the resolution of obstructive sleep apnea syndrome: a case report. *J Chiropr Med, 10*(2), 118-25. doi: 10.1016/j.jcm.2010.12.003

Gangloff, A., Bergeron, J., Lemieux, I., Tremblay, A., Poirier, P., Alméras, N. & Després, J. (2020). Relationships between circulating 25(OH) vitamin D, leptin levels and visceral adipose tissue volume: results from a 1-year lifestyle intervention program in men with visceral obesity. *Int J Obes (Lond), 44*(2), 280-288. doi: 10.1038/s41366-019-0347-7

Ganguly, K., Levänen, B., Palmberg, L., Åkesson, A. & Lindén, A. (2018). Cadmium in tobacco smokers: a neglected link to lung disease? *Eur Respir Rev, 27*(147), 170122. doi: 10.1183/16000617.0122-2017

Gangwisch, J., Heymsfield, S., Boden-Albala, B., Buijs, R., Kreier, F., Pickering, T., … Malaspina, D. (2006). Short sleep duration as a risk factor for hypertension: analyses of the first National Health and Nutrition Examination Survey. *Hypertension, 47*(5), 833-9. doi: 10.1161/01.HYP.0000217362.34748.e0

Gariazzo, C., Gasparrini, A. & Marinaccio, A. (2023). Asbestos Consumption and Malignant Mesothelioma Mortality Trends in the Major User Countries. *Ann Glob Health, 89*(1), 11. doi: 10.5334/aogh.4012

Gaspari, L., Soyer-Gobillard, M., Rincheval, N., Paris, F., Kalfa, N., Hamamah, S. & Sultan, C. (2023). Birth outcomes in DES children and grandchildren: A multigenerational national cohort study on informative families. *Int J Environ Res Public Health, 20*(3), 2542. doi: 10.3390/ijerph20032542

Gehlert, S. & Clanton, M., On behalf of the shift work

and breast cancer strategic advisory group. (2020). Shift work and breast cancer. *Int J Environ Res Public Health, 17*(24), 9544. doi: 10.3390/ijerph17249544

Gencer, B., Djousse, L., Al-Ramady, O., Cook, N., Manson, J. & Albert, C. (2021). Effect of Long-Term Marine ω-3 Fatty Acids Supplementation on the Risk of Atrial Fibrillation in Randomized Controlled Trials of Cardiovascular Outcomes: A Systematic Review and Meta-Analysis. *Circulation, 144*(25), 1981-1990. doi: 10.1161/CIRCULATIONAHA.121.055654

Gesch, C., Hammond, S., Hampson, S., Eves, A. & Crowder, M. (2002). Influence of supplementary vitamins, minerals and essential fatty acids on the antisocial behaviour of young adult prisoners. Randomised, placebo-controlled trial. *Br J Psychiatry, 181*, 22-8. doi: 10.1192/bjp.181.1.22

Ghahremani, M., Smith, E., Chen, H., Creese, B., Goodarzi, Z. & Ismail, Z. (2023). Vitamin D supplementation and incident dementia: Effects of sex, *APOE*, and baseline cognitive status. *Alzheimers Dement (Amst), 15*(1), e12404. doi: 10.1002/dad2.12404

Ghiadoni, L. & Bernini, G. (2016). Cholecalciferol treatment downregulates renin-angiotensin system and improves endothelial function in essential hypertensive patients with hypovitaminosid D. *J Hypertens, 34*(11), 2199-205. doi: 10.1097/HJH.0000000000001072

Ghiadoni, L., Donald, A., Cropley, M., Mullen, M., Oakley, G., Taylor, M., … Deanfield, J. (2000). Mental stress induces transient endothelial dysfunction in humans. *Circulation, 102*(20), 2473-8. doi: 10.1161/01.cir.102.20.2473

Glibowski, P. (2020). Organic food and health. *Rocz Panstw Zakl Hig, 71*(2), 131-136. doi: 10.32394/rpzh.2020.0110

Gohil, A. & Hannon, T. (2018). Poor sleep and obesity: Concurrent epidemics in adolescent youth. *Front Endocrinol (Lausanne), 9*, 364. doi: 10.3389/fendo.2018.00364

Goldstein, M., Mascitelli, L. & Pezzetta, F. (2008). Do statins prevent or promote cancer? Curr Oncol. 2008 Apr;15(2):76-7. doi: 10.3747/co.v15i2.235

Golomb, B., Stattin, H. & Mednick, S. (2000). Low cholesterol and violent crime. *J Psychiatr Res, 34*(4-5), 301-9. doi: 10.1016/s0022-3956(00)00024-8

Gonçalves, T., Gonçalves, S., Guarnieri, A., Risegato, R., Guimarães MP, de Freitas DC, … Parrillo, E. (2020). Prevalence of obesity and hypovitaminosis D in elderly with severe acute respiratory syndrome coronavirus 2 (SARS-CoV-2). *Clin Nutr ESPEN, 40*, 110-114. doi: 10.1016/j.clnesp.2020.10.008

Gong, J., Shen, Y., Shan, W., & He, Y. (2018). The association between MTHFR polymorphism and cervical cancer. *Sci Rep, 8*(1), 7244. doi: 10.1038/s41598-018-25726-9

Gonsioroski, A., Mourikes, V. & Flaws, J. (2020). Endocrine disruptors in water and their effects on the reproductive system. *Int J Mol Sci, 21*(6), 1929. doi: 10.3390/ijms21061929

Gøtzsche, P. & Olsen, O. (2000) Is screening for breast cancer with mammography justifiable? *Lancet, 355*(9198), 129-34. doi: 10.1016/S0140-6736(99)06065-1

Gøtzsche, P. (2014). Our prescription drugs kill us in large numbers. *Pol Arch Med Wewn, 124*(11), 628-34. doi: 10.20452/pamw.2503

Gøtzsche, P. (2015). Mammography screening is harmful and should be abandoned. *J R Soc Med, 108*(9), 341-5. doi: 10.1177/0141076815602452

Gøtzsche, P. (2017). Rapid Response: Antidepressants increase the risk of suicide, violence and homicide at all ages. *BMJ, 358,* j3697. doi: 10.1136/bmj.j3697

Grandjean, P. (2019). Developmental fluoride neurotoxicity: an updated review. *Environ Health, 18*(1), 110. doi: 10.1186/s12940-019-0551-x

Grant, W. (2007). A meta-analysis of second cancers after a diagnosis of nonmelanoma skin cancer: additional evidence that solar ultraviolet-B irradiance reduces the risk of internal cancers. *J Steroid Biochem Mol Biol, 103*(3-5), 668-74. doi: 10.1016/j.jsbmb.2006.12.030

Grant, W. (2007). A meta-analysis of second cancers after a diagnosis of nonmelanoma skin cancer: additional evidence that solar ultraviolet-B irradiance reduces the risk of internal cancers. *J Steroid Biochem Mol Biol, 103*(3-5), 668-74. doi: 10.1016/j.jsbmb.2006.12.030

Gröber, U., Schmidt, J. & Kisters, K. (2015). Magnesium in prevention and therapy. *Nutrients, 7*(9), 8199-226. doi: 10.3390/nu7095388

Gross, L., Li, L., Ford, E. & Liu, S. (2004). Increased consumption of refined carbohydrates and the epidemic of type 2 diabetes in the United States: an ecologic assessment. *Am J Clin Nutr, 79*(5), 774-9. doi: 10.1093/ajcn/79.5.774

Guan, Y., Dai, P. & Wang, H. (2020). Effects of

vitamin C supplementation on essential hypertension: A systematic review and meta-analysis. *Medicine (Baltimore), 99*(8), e19274. doi: 10.1097/MD.0000000000019274

Guo, H., Zhang, R., Zhang, P., Chen, Z., Hua, Y., Huang, X. & Li, X. (2023). Association of proton pump inhibitors with gastric and colorectal cancer risk: A systematic review and meta-analysis. *Front Pharmacol, 14*, 1129948. doi: 10.3389/fphar.2023.1129948

Gupta, R., Gangoliya, S. & Singh, N. (2015) Reduction of phytic acid and enhancement of bioavailable micronutrients in food grains. *J Food Sci Technol, 52*(2), 676-84. doi: 10.1007/s13197-013-0978-y

Gylling, H., Hallikainen, M., Pihlajamäki, J., Simonen, P., Kuusisto, J., Laakso, M. & Miettinen, T. (2010). Insulin sensitivity regulates cholesterol metabolism to a greater extent than obesity: lessons from the METSIM Study. *J Lipid Res, 51*(8), 2422-7. doi: 10.1194/jlr.P006619

Györéné, K., Varga, A. & Lugasi, A. (2006). Az ökológiai (bio) és konvencionális termesztésu növényi élelmiszerek beltartalmának, táplálkozási értékének összehasonlítása [A comparison of chemical composition and nutritional value of organically and conventionally grown plant derived foods]. *Orv Hetil,*

147(43), 2081-90. Hungarian

Habib, A., Katz, M. & Redberg, R. (2022). Statins for primary cardiovascular disease prevention: Time to curb our enthusiasm. *JAMA Intern Med, 182*(10), 1021-1024. doi: 10.1001/jamainternmed.2022.3204

Hagele, T., Mazerik, J., Gregory, A., Kaufman, B., Magalang, U., Kuppusamy, M., … Parinandi, N. (2007). Mercury activates vascular endothelial cell phospholipase D through thiols and oxidative stress. *Int J Toxicol, 26*(1), 57-69. doi: 10.1080/10915810601120509

Hales, C. & Barker, D. (2001). The thrifty phenotype hypothesis. *Br Med Bull, 60*, 5-20. doi: 10.1093/bmb/60.1.5

Hall, R., Friedman, S., Sorrentino, R., Lapchenko, M., Marcus, A. & Ellis, R. (2019), The myth of school shooters and psychotropic medications. *Behav Sci Law, 37*(5):540-558. doi: 10.1002/bsl.2429

Hamilton, G. & Joosten, S. (2017). Obstructive sleep apnoea and obesity. *Aust Fam Physician, 46*(7), 460-463.

Hammarsten, J. & Högstedt, B. (2005). Hyperinsulinaemia: a prospective risk factor for lethal clinical prostate cancer. *Eur J Cancer, 41*(18), 2887-95.

doi: 10.1016/j.ejca.2005.09.003

Harris, J., Pomeranz, J., Lobstein, T. & Brownell, K. (2009). A crisis in the marketplace: how food marketing contributes to childhood obesity and what can be done. *Annu Rev Public Health, 30*, 211-25. doi: 10.1146/annurev.publhealth.031308.100304

Hasrat, N. & Al-Yassen, A. (2023). The Relationship Between Acne Vulgaris and Insulin Resistance. *Cureus, 15*(1), e34241. doi: 10.7759/cureus.34241

Hathcock, J. & Shao, A. (2006). Risk assessment for coenzyme Q10 (Ubiquinone*). Regul Toxicol Pharmacol, 45*(3), 282-8. doi: 10.1016/j.yrtph.2006.05.006

Havel, P. (2004). A scientific review: the role of chromium in insulin resistance. *Diabetes Educ, Suppl*, 2-14

Haverinen, E., Fernandez, M., Mustieles, V. & Tolonen, H. (2021). Metabolic syndrome and endocrine disrupting chemicals: An overview of exposure and health effects. *Int J Environ Res Public Health, 18*(24), 13047. doi: 10.3390/ijerph182413047

Hawley, J. (2004). Exercise as a therapeutic intervention for the prevention and treatment of insulin resistance. *Diabetes Metab Res Rev, 20*(5), 383-93. doi:

10.1002/dmrr.505

Hays, J., Gorman, R. & Shakir, K. (2002). Results of use of metformin and replacement of starch with saturated fat in diets of patients with type 2 diabetes. *Endocr Pract, 8*(3), 177-83. doi: 10.4158/EP.8.3.177

Heller, S. & Moy, L. (2019). MRI breast screening revisited. *J Magn Reson Imaging, 49*(5), 1212-1221. doi: 10.1002/jmri.26547

Helte, E., Donat Vargas, C., Kippler, M., Wolk, A., Michaëlsson, K., Åkesson, A. (2021). Fluoride in drinking water, diet, and urine in relation to bone mineral density and fracture incidence in postmenopausal women. *Environ Health Perspect, 129*(4), 47005. doi: 10.1289/EHP7404

Henein, M., Vancheri, S., Longo, G. & Vancheri, F. (2022). The role of inflammation in cardiovascular disease. *Int J Mol Sci, 23*(21), 12906. doi: 10.3390/ijms232112906

Hepworth, S., Schoemaker, M., Muir, K., Swerdlow, A., van Tongeren, M. & McKinney, P. (2006). Mobile phone use and risk of glioma in adults: case-control study. *BMJ, 332*(7546), 883-7. doi: 10.1136/bmj.38720.687975.55

Hercberg, S., Ezzedine, K., Guinot, C., Preziosi, P.,

Galan, P., Bertrais, S., … Malvy, D. (2007). Antioxidant supplementation increases the risk of skin cancers in women but not in men. *J Nutr, 137*(9), 2098-105. doi: 10.1093/jn/137.9.2098

Hillbrand, M., Waite, B., Miller, D., Spitz, R. & Lingswiler, V. (2000). Serum cholesterol concentrations and mood states in violent psychiatric patients: an experience sampling study. *J Behav Med, 23*(6), 519-29. doi: 10.1023/a:1005551418922

Ho, S., Woodford, K., Kukuljan, S. & Pal, S. (2014). Comparative effects of A1 versus A2 beta-casein on gastrointestinal measures: a blinded randomised cross-over pilot study. *Eur J Clin Nutr, 68*(9), 994-1000. doi: 10.1038/ejcn.2014.127

Holl, M. & Allen, L. (1987). Sucrose ingestion, insulin response and mineral metabolism in humans. *J Nutr, 117*(7), 1229-33. doi: 10.1093/jn/117.7.1229

Holtorf, K. (2009). The bioidentical hormone debate: are bioidentical hormones (estradiol, estriol, and progesterone) safer or more efficacious than commonly used synthetic versions in hormone replacement therapy? *Postgrad Med, 121*(1), 73-85. doi: 10.3810/pgm.2009.01.1949

Hoover, D, & Milich, R. (1994). Effects of sugar ingestion expectancies on mother-child interactions. *J*

Abnorm Child Psychol, 22(4), 501-15. doi: 10.1007/BF02168088

Horne, B., May, H., Anderson, J., Kfoury, A., Bailey, B., McClure, B., … Muhlestein, J.; Intermountain Heart Collaborative Study. (2008). Usefulness of routine periodic fasting to lower risk of coronary artery disease in patients undergoing coronary angiography. *Am J Cardiol, 102*(7), 814-819. doi: 10.1016/j.amjcard.2008.05.021

Horsten, M., Wamala, S., Vingerhoets, A. & Orth-Gomer, K. (1997). Depressive symptoms, social support, and lipid profile in healthy middle-aged women. *Psychosom Med, 59*(5), 521-8. Doi: 10.1097/00006842-199709000-00009

Hosokawa, R., Tomozawa, R., Fujimoto, M., Anzai., S, Sato, M., Tazoe, H. & Katsura, T. (2022). Association between sleep habits and behavioral problems in early adolescence: a descriptive study. *BMC Psychol, 10*(1), 254. doi: 10.1186/s40359-022-00958-7

Houston, M. (2011). The role of magnesium in hypertension and cardiovascular disease. *J Clin Hypertens (Greenwich), 13*(11), 843-7. doi: 10.1111/j.1751-7176.2011.00538.x

Høyer, A., Jørgensen, T., Brock, J. & Grandjean, P.

(2000). Organochlorine exposure and breast cancer survival. *J Clin Epidemiol, 53*(3), 323-30. doi: 10.1016/s0895-4356(99)00165-1

Hughes, M., van der Pols, J., Marks, G. & Green, A. (2006). Food intake and risk of squamous cell carcinoma of the skin in a community: the Nambour skin cancer cohort study. *Int J Cancer, 119*(8), 1953-60. doi: 10.1002/ijc.22061

Huseini, H., Larijani, B., Heshmat, R., Fakhrzadeh, H., Radjabipour, B., Toliat, T. & Raza, M. (2006). The efficacy of Silybum marianum (L.) Gaertn. (silymarin) in the treatment of type II diabetes: a randomized, double-blind, placebo-controlled, clinical trial. *Phytother Res, 20*(12), 1036-9. doi: 10.1002/ptr.1988

Ilich, J., Brownbill, R., Tamborini, L., Crncevic-Orlic, Z. (2002). To drink or not to drink: how are alcohol, caffeine and past smoking related to bone mineral density in elderly women? *J Am Coll Nutr, 21*(6), 536-44. doi: 10.1080/07315724.2002.10719252

Imamura, F., O'Connor, L., Ye, Z., Mursu, J., Hayashino, Y., Bhupathiraju, S. & Forouhi, N. (2015). Consumption of sugar sweetened beverages, artificially sweetened beverages, and fruit juice and incidence of type 2 diabetes: systematic review, meta-analysis, and estimation of population attributable fraction. *BMJ,*

351, h3576. doi: 10.1136/bmj.h3576

Ioannidis, J. (2005) Why most published research findings are false. *PLoS Med, 2*(8), e124. doi: 10.1371/journal.pmed.0020124

Jahrami, H, Faris, M., I Janahi, A., I Janahi, M., Abdelrahim, D., Madkour, M., … Bahammam, A. (2021). Does four-week consecutive, dawn-to-sunset intermittent fasting during Ramadan affect cardiometabolic risk factors in healthy adults? A systematic review, meta-analysis, and meta-regression. *Nutr Metab Cardiovasc Dis, 31*(8), 2273-2301. doi: 10.1016/j.numecd.2021.05.002

Janoutová, J., Machaczka, O., Zatloukalová, A. & Janout, V. (2022). Is Alzheimer's disease a type 3 diabetes? A review. *Cent Eur J Public Health, 30*(3), 139-143. doi: 10.21101/cejph.a7238

Järup, L. (2003). Hazards of heavy metal contamination. *Br Med Bull, 68*, 167-82. doi: 10.1093/bmb/ldg032

Jarvill-Taylor, K., Anderson, R. & Graves, D. (2001). A hydroxychalcone derived from cinnamon functions as a mimetic for insulin in 3T3-L1 adipocytes. J Am Coll Nutr. 2001 Aug;20(4):327-36. doi: 10.1080/07315724.2001.10719053

Jeong, H, Park, K., Lee, M., Yang, D., Kim, S. & Lee, S. (2017). Vitamin D and hypertension. *Electrolyte Blood Press, 15*(1), 1-11. doi: 10.5049/EBP.2017.15.1.1

Jianqin, S., Leiming, X., Lu, X., Yelland, G., Ni, J. & Clarke, A. (2016). Effects of milk containing only A2 beta casein versus milk containing both A1 and A2 beta casein proteins on gastrointestinal physiology, symptoms of discomfort, and cognitive behavior of people with self-reported intolerance to traditional cows' milk. *Nutr J, 15*, 35. doi: 10.1186/s12937-016-0147-z

Johnson, M., Kenney, N., Stoica, A., Hilakivi-Clarke, L., Singh, B., Chepko, G., … Martin, M. (2003). Cadmium mimics the in vivo effects of estrogen in the uterus and mammary gland. *Nat Med, 9*(8), 1081-4. doi: 10.1038/nm902

Jones, H., Borges, M., Carnegie, R., Mongan, D., Rogers, P., Lewis, S., … Zammit, S. (2021). Associations between plasma fatty acid concentrations and schizophrenia: a two-sample Mendelian randomisation study. *Lancet Psychiatry, 8*(12), 1062-1070. doi: 10.1016/S2215-0366(21)00286-8

Joseph, M., Tincopa, M., Walden, P., Jackson, E., Conte, M. & Rubenfire, M. (2019). The impact of structured exercise programs on metabolic syndrome and its components: A systematic review. *Diabetes Metab Syndr Obes, 12*, 2395-2404. doi: 10.2147/DMSO.S211776

Ju, W., Li, X., Li, Z., Wu, G., Fu, X., Yang, X.., … Gao, X. (2017). The effect of selenium supplementation on coronary heart disease: A systematic review and meta-analysis of randomized controlled trials. *J Trace Elem Med Biol, 44*, 8-16. doi: 10.1016/j.jtemb.2017.04.009

Kalfa, N., Paris, F., Soyer-Gobillard, M., Daures, J. & Sultan, C. (2011). Prevalence of hypospadias in grandsons of women exposed to diethylstilbestrol during pregnancy: a multigenerational national cohort study. *Fertil Steril, 95*(8), 2574-7. doi: 10.1016/j.fertnstert.2011.02.047

Kaplan, N. (1989). The deadly quartet. Upper-body obesity, glucose intolerance, hypertriglyceridemia, and hypertension. *Arch Intern Med, 149*(7), 1514-20. doi: 10.1001/archinte.149.7.1514

Karatzi, K., Papamichael, C., Karatzis, E., Papaioannou, T., Voidonikola, P., Lekakis, J. & Zampelas, A. (2007). Acute smoking induces endothelial dysfunction in healthy smokers. Is this reversible by red wine's antioxidant constituents? *J Am*

Coll Nutr, 26(1), 10-5. doi: 10.1080/07315724.2007.10719580

Karlsson, B., Knutsson, A. & Lindahl, B. (2001). Is there an association between shift work and having a metabolic syndrome? Results from a population based study of 27,485 people. *Occup Environ Med, 58*(11), 747-52. doi: 10.1136/oem.58.11.747

Katalinic, A. & Rawal, R. (2008). Decline in breast cancer incidence after decrease in utilisation of hormone replacement therapy. *Breast Cancer Res Treat, 107*(3), 427-30. doi: 10.1007/s10549-007-9566-z

Kavalipati, N., Shah, J., Ramakrishan, A. & Vasnawala, H. (2015). Pleiotropic effects of statins. *Indian J Endocrinol Metab, 19*(5), 554-62. doi: 10.4103/2230-8210.163106

Kearns, C., Schmidt, L. & Glantz, S. (2016) Sugar industry and coronary heart disease research: A historical analysis of internal industry documents. *JAMA Intern Med, 176*(11), 1680-1685. doi: 10.1001/jamainternmed.2016.5394

Kekwick, A. & Pawan, G. (1956). Calorie intake in relation to body-weight changes in the obese. *Lancet, 271*(6935), 155-61. doi: 10.1016/s0140-6736(56)91691-9

Kemmler, W., Engelke, K., Weineck, J., Hensen, J. & Kalender, W. (2003). The Erlangen Fitness Osteoporosis Prevention Study: a controlled exercise trial in early postmenopausal women with low bone density-first-year results. *Arch Phys Med Rehabil, 84*(5), 673-82. doi: 10.1016/s0003-9993(02)04908-0

Kerlikowske, K., Salzmann, P., Phillips, K., Cauley, J. & Cummings, S. (1999). Continuing screening mammography in women aged 70 to 79 years: impact on life expectancy and cost-effectiveness. *JAMA, 282*(22), 2156-63. doi: 10.1001/jama.282.22.2156

Khan, A., Safdar, M., Ali Khan, M., Khattak, K. & Anderson, R. (2003). Cinnamon improves glucose and lipids of people with type 2 diabetes. *Diabetes Care, 26*(12), 3215-8. doi: 10.2337/diacare.26.12.3215

Khan, S., Lone, A., Khan, M., Virani, S., Blumenthal, R., Nasir, K., … Bhatt, D. (2021). Effect of omega-3 fatty acids on cardiovascular outcomes: A systematic review and meta-analysis. *EClinicalMedicine, 38*, 100997. doi: 10.1016/j.eclinm.2021.100997

Kim, J., Montagnani, M., Koh, K. & Quon, M. (2006). Reciprocal relationships between insulin resistance and endothelial dysfunction: molecular and pathophysiological mechanisms. *Circulation, 113*(15), 1888-904. doi:

10.1161/CIRCULATIONAHA.105.563213

Kim, Y. & Myint, A. (2004). Clinical application of low serum cholesterol as an indicator for suicide risk in major depression. *J Affect Disord, 81*(2), 161-6. doi: 10.1016/S0165-0327(03)00166-6

Kirkham, S., Akilen, R., Sharma, S. & Tsiami, A. (2009). The potential of cinnamon to reduce blood glucose levels in patients with type 2 diabetes and insulin resistance. *Diabetes Obes Metab, 11*(12), 1100-13. doi: 10.1111/j.1463-1326.2009.01094.x

Klip, H., Verloop, J., van Gool, J., Koster, M., Burger, C. & van Leeuwen, F.; OMEGA Project Group. (2002). Hypospadias in sons of women exposed to diethylstilbestrol in utero: a cohort study. *Lancet, 359*(9312), 1102-7. doi: 10.1016/S0140-6736(02)08152-7

Kohn, L., Corrigan, J. & Donaldson, M. (editors) (2009). Institute of Medicine (US) Committee on Quality of Health Care in America. To Err is Human: Building a Safer Health System. Washington (DC): National Academies Press (US).

Kostis, J. & Dobrzynski, J. (2019). Statins and erectile dysfunction. *World J Mens Health, 37*(1), 1-3. doi: 10.5534/wjmh.180015

Krawinkel, M, & Keding, G. (2006). Bitter gourd (Momordica Charantia): A dietary approach to hyperglycemia. *Nutr Rev, 64*(7 Pt 1), 331-7. doi: 10.1301/nr.2006.jul.331-337

KrishnaRaju, A., Somepalli, V., Thanawala, S. & Shah, R. (2023). Efficacy and anti-inflammatory activity of ashwagandha sustained-release formulation on depression and anxiety induced by chronic unpredictable stress: in vivo and in vitro studies. *J Exp Pharmacol, 15*, 291-305. doi: 10.2147/JEP.S407906

Kristensen, M., Christensen, P. & Hallas, J. (2015). The effect of statins on average survival in randomised trials, an analysis of end point postponement. *BMJ Open, 5*(9), e007118. doi: 10.1136/bmjopen-2014-007118

Krousel-Wood, M., Muntner, P., He, J. & Whelton, P. (2004). Primary prevention of essential hypertension. *Med Clin North Am, 88*(1), 223-38. doi: 10.1016/s0025-7125(03)00126-3

Krumholz, H., Seeman, T., Merrill, S., Mendes de Leon, C., Vaccarino, V., Silverman, D., … Berkman, L. (1994). Lack of association between cholesterol and coronary heart disease mortality and morbidity and all-cause mortality in persons older than 70 years. JAMA. 1994 Nov 2;272(17):1335-40.

Kuo, L., Kitlinska, J., Tilan, J., Li, L., Baker, S., Johnson, M., … Zukowska, Z. (2007). Neuropeptide Y acts directly in the periphery on fat tissue and mediates stress-induced obesity and metabolic syndrome. *Nat Med, 13*(7), 803-11. doi: 10.1038/nm1611

Kuria, A., Fang, X., Li, M., Han, H., He, J., Aaseth, J., & Cao, Y. (2020). Does dietary intake of selenium protect against cancer? A systematic review and meta-analysis of population-based prospective studies. *Crit Rev Food Sci Nutr, 60*(4), 684-694. doi: 10.1080/10408398.2018.1548427

Kyle, U & Pichard, C. (2006). The Dutch Famine of 1944-1945: a pathophysiological model of long-term consequences of wasting disease. *Curr Opin Clin Nutr Metab Care, 9*(4), 388-94. doi: 10.1097/01.mco.0000232898.74415.42

Laguna, J., Alegret, M., Cofán, M., Sánchez-Tainta, A., Díaz-López, A., Martínez-González, M., … Ros, E. (2021). Simple sugar intake and cancer incidence, cancer mortality and all-cause mortality: A cohort study from the PREDIMED trial. *Clin Nutr, 40*(10), 5269-5277. doi: 10.1016/j.clnu.2021.07.031

Lahkola, A., Auvinen, A., Raitanen, J., Schoemaker, M., Christensen, H., Feychting, M., … Salminen, T. (2007). Mobile phone use and risk of glioma in 5 North

European countries. *Int J Cancer, 120*(8), 1769-75. doi: 10.1002/ijc.22503

Lamat, H., Sauvant-Rochat, M., Tauveron, I., Bagheri, R., Ugbolue, U., Maqdasi, S., … Dutheil, F. (2022). Metabolic syndrome and pesticides: A systematic review and meta-analysis. *Environ Pollut, 305*, 119288. doi: 10.1016/j.envpol.2022.119288

Landrigan, P. & Straif, K. (2021). Aspartame and cancer - new evidence for causation. *Environ Health, 20*(1), 42. doi: 10.1186/s12940-021-00725-y

Langsjoen, P. & Langsjoen, A. (2003). The clinical use of HMG CoA-reductase inhibitors and the associated depletion of coenzyme Q10. A review of animal and human publications. *Biofactors, 18*(1-4), 101-11. doi: 10.1002/biof.5520180212

Lanou, A., Berkow, S. & Barnard, N. (2005). Calcium, dairy products, and bone health in children and young adults: a reevaluation of the evidence. *Pediatrics, 115*(3), 736-43. doi: 10.1542/peds.2004-0548

Lappe, J., Travers-Gustafson, D., Davies, K., Recker, R. & Heaney, R. (2007). Vitamin D and calcium supplementation reduces cancer risk: results of a randomized trial. *Am J Clin Nutr, 85*(6), 1586-91. doi: 10.1093/ajcn/85.6.1586. Erratum in: Am J Clin Nutr.

2008 Mar;87(3):794

Larson, E., Wang, L., Bowen, J., McCormick, W., Teri, L., Crane, P. & Kukull, W. (2006). Exercise is associated with reduced risk for incident dementia among persons 65 years of age and older. *Ann Intern Med, 144*(2), 73-81. doi: 10.7326/0003-4819-144-2-200601170-00004

La Vecchia, C., Franceschi, S., Dolara, P., Bidoli, E. & Barbone, F. (1993). Refined-sugar intake and the risk of colorectal cancer in humans. *Int J Cancer, 55*(3), 386-9. doi: 10.1002/ijc.2910550308

Lawlor, D., Smith, G. & Ebrahim, S. (2004). Hyperinsulinaemia and increased risk of breast cancer: findings from the British Women's Heart and Health Study. *Cancer Causes Control, 15*(3), 267-75. doi: 10.1023/B:CACO.0000024225

Leatherdale, B., Panesar, R., Singh, G., Atkins, T., Bailey, C. & Bignell, A. (1981). Improvement in glucose tolerance due to Momordica charantia (karela). *Br Med J (Clin Res Ed), 282*(6279), 1823-4. doi: 10.1136/bmj.282.6279.1823

Le Roy, T., Lécuyer, E., Chassaing, B., Rhimi, M., Lhomme, M., Boudebbouze, S., … Lesnik, P. (2019). The intestinal microbiota regulates host cholesterol homeostasis. *BMC Biol, 17*(1), 94. doi:

10.1186/s12915-019-0715-8

Levine, H., Jørgensen, N., Martino-Andrade, A., Mendiola, J., Weksler-Derri, D., Mindlis, I., … Swan, S. (21017). Temporal trends in sperm count: a systematic review and meta-regression analysis. *Hum Reprod Update, 23*(6), 646-659. doi: 10.1093/humupd/dmx022

Levitt Katz, L., Swami, S., Abraham, M., Murphy, K., Jawad, A., McKnight-Menci, H. & Berkowitz, R. (2005). Neuropsychiatric disorders at the presentation of type 2 diabetes mellitus in children. *Pediatr Diabetes, 6*(2), 84-9. doi: 10.1111/j.1399-543X.2005.00105.x

Li, H., Sureda, A., Devkota, H., Pittalà, V., Barreca, D., Silva, A., … Nabavi, S. (2020). Curcumin, the golden spice in treating cardiovascular diseases. *Biotechnol Adv, 38*, 107343. doi: 10.1016/j.biotechadv.2019.01.010

Li, Y. & Xu, Z. (2021). Effects of melatonin supplementation on insulin levels and insulin resistance: A systematic review and meta-analysis of randomized controlled trials. *Horm Metab Res, 53*(9), 616-624. doi: 10.1055/a-1544-8181

Li, Y., Kong, J., Wei, M., Chen, Z., Liu, S. & Cao, L.

(2002). 1,25-Dihydroxyvitamin D(3) is a negative endocrine regulator of the renin-angiotensin system. *J Clin Invest, 110*(2), 229-38. doi: 10.1172/JCI15219

Li, Y., Liang, C., Slemenda, C., Ji, R., Sun, S., Cao, J., … Johnston, C. Jr. (2001). Effect of long-term exposure to fluoride in drinking water on risks of bone fractures. J Bone Miner Res. 2001 May;16(5):932-9. doi: 10.1359/jbmr.2001.16.5.932

Li, Y., Yang, A., Wang, W., Wang, Z., Wang, Z., Su, X., … Hao, M. (2020). Folic acid intake and folate status and risk of cervical cancer: A systematic review and meta-analysis from 20 independent case-control studies and 4 RCTs. *Curr Dev Nutr, 4*(Suppl 2), 330. doi: 10.1093/cdn/nzaa044_029

Liang, Y., Vetrano, D. & Qiu. C. (2017). Serum total cholesterol and risk of cardiovascular and non-cardiovascular mortality in old age: a population-based study. *BMC Geriatr, 17*(1), 294. doi: 10.1186/s12877-017-0685-z

Liao, J., Xiong, Q., Yin, Y., Ling, Z. & Chen, S. (2022). The effects of fish oil on cardiovascular diseases: Systematical evaluation and recent advance. *Front Cardiovasc Med, 8*, 802306. doi: 10.3389/fcvm.2021.802306

Lien, L., Lien, N., Heyerdahl, S., Thoresen, M. &

Bjertness, E. (2006). Consumption of soft drinks and hyperactivity, mental distress, and conduct problems among adolescents in Oslo, Norway. *Am J Public Health, 96*(10), 1815-20. doi: 10.2105/AJPH.2004.059477

Lincoff, A., Nicholls, S., Riesmeyer, J., Barter, P., Brewer, H., Fox, K., … Nissen, S.; ACCELERATE Investigators. (2017). Evacetrapib and cardiovascular outcomes in high-risk vascular disease. *N Engl J Med, 376*(20),1933-1942. doi: 10.1056/NEJMoa1609581

Llaha, F., Gil-Lespinard, M., Unal, P., de Villasante, I., Castañeda, J. & Zamora-Ros, R. (2021). Consumption of Sweet Beverages and Cancer Risk. A Systematic Review and Meta-Analysis of Observational Studies. *Nutrients, 13*(2), 516. doi: 10.3390/nu13020516

Loke, K. (2014). Early influences in childhood obesity--implications for adult metabolic disease. *Ann Acad Med Singap, 43*(1), 57-8.

Longo, V., Di Tano, M., Mattson, M. & Guidi, N. (2021). Intermittent and periodic fasting, longevity and disease. *Nat Aging, 1*(1), 47-59. doi: 10.1038/s43587-020-00013-3

Lowenthal, R., Tuck, D. & Bray, I. (2007). Residential

exposure to electric power transmission lines and risk of lymphoproliferative and myeloproliferative disorders: a case-control study. *Intern Med J, 37*(9), 614-9. doi: 10.1111/j.1445-5994.2007.01389.x

Lucienne, J., Tynes, T. & Andersen, A. (2001). Risk of breast cancer among Norwegian women with visual impairment. *Br J Cancer, 84*(3), 397-9. doi: 10.1054/bjoc.2000.1617

Ludwig, D., Peterson, K. & Gortmaker, S. (2001). Relation between consumption of sugar-sweetened drinks and childhood obesity: a prospective, observational analysis. *Lancet, 357*(9255), 505-8. doi: 10.1016/S0140-6736(00)04041-1

Lustberg, M. & Silbergeld, E. (2002). Blood lead levels and mortality. *Arch Intern Med, 162*(21), 2443-9. doi: 10.1001/archinte.162.21.2443

MacMahon, S., Neal, B. & Rodgers, A. (2005). Hypertension--time to move on. *Lancet, 365*(9464), 1108-9. doi: 10.1016/S0140-6736(05)71148-X

Makary, M. & Daniel, M. (2016). Medical error-the third leading cause of death in the US. *BMJ, 353*, i2139. doi: 10.1136/bmj.i2139

Maksimović, Z., Rsumović, M., Jović, V., Kosanović, M. & Jovanović, T. (1998). Selenium in soil, grass, and human serum in the Zlatibor mountain area (Serbia): geomedical aspects. *J Environ Pathol Toxicol Oncol, 17*(3-4), 221-7.

Malhotra, A., Redberg, R. & Meier, P. (2017). Saturated fat does not clog the arteries: coronary heart disease is a chronic inflammatory condition, the risk of which can be effectively reduced from healthy lifestyle interventions. *Br J Sports Med, 51*(15), 1111-1112. doi: 10.1136/bjsports-2016-097285

Mancini, M., Hémon, D., de Crouy-Chanel, P., Guldner, L., Faure, L., Clavel, J. & Goujon, S. (2023). Association between residential proximity to viticultural areas and childhood acute leukemia risk in mainland France: GEOCAP case-control study, 2006-2013. *Environ Health Perspect, 131*(10), 107008. doi: 10.1289/EHP12634

Mann, U., Shiff, B. & Patel, P. (2020). Reasons for worldwide decline in male fertility. *Curr Opin Urol, 30*(3), 296-301. doi: 10.1097/MOU.0000000000000745

Mansi, I., Sumithran, P. & Kinaan, M. (2023). Risk of diabetes with statins. *BMJ, 381*, e071727. doi: 10.1136/bmj-2022-071727

Mansi, I., Chansard, M., Lingvay, I., Zhang, S., Halm, E. & Alvarez, C. (2021). Association of statin therapy initiation with diabetes progression: A retrospective matched-cohort study. *JAMA Intern Med, 181*(12), 1562-1574. doi: 10.1001/jamainternmed.2021.5714

Marchesini, G., Marzocchi, R., Agostini, F. & Bugianesi, E. (2005). Nonalcoholic fatty liver disease and the metabolic syndrome. *Curr Opin Lipidol, 16*(4), 421-7. doi: 10.1097/01.mol.0000174153.53683.f2

Marchioli, R., Levantesi, G., Macchia, A., Maggioni, A., Marfisi, R., Silletta, M., … Valagussa F; GISSI-Prevenzione Investigators. (2005). Antiarrhythmic mechanisms of n-3 PUFA and the results of the GISSI-Prevenzione trial. *J Membr Biol, 206*(2), 117-28. doi: 10.1007/s00232-005-0788-x

Marcus, C., Nyberg, G., Nordenfelt, A., Karpmyr, M., Kowalski, J. & Ekelund, U. (2009). A 4-year, cluster-randomized, controlled childhood obesity prevention study: STOPP. *Int J Obes (Lond), 33*(4), 408-17. doi: 10.1038/ijo.2009.38

Maresz, K. (2015). Proper Calcium Use: Vitamin K2 as a Promoter of Bone and Cardiovascular Health. *Integr Med (Encinitas), 14*(1), 34-9

Mazidi, M., Katsiki, N., George, E. & Banach, M. (2020). Tomato and lycopene consumption is inversely associated with total and cause-specific mortality: a population-based cohort study, on behalf of the

International Lipid Expert Panel (ILEP). *Br J Nutr, 124*(12), 1303-1310. doi: 10.1017/S0007114519002150

McCann, D., Barrett, A., Cooper, A., Crumpler, D., Dalen, L., Grimshaw, K., … Stevenson, J. (2007). Food additives and hyperactive behaviour in 3-year-old and 8/9-year-old children in the community: a randomised, double-blinded, placebo-controlled trial. *Lancet, 370*(9598), 1560-7. doi: 10.1016/S0140-6736(07)61306-3

Medical Research Council Working Party. (1985) MRC trial of treatment of mild hypertension: principal results. *Br Med J (Clin Res Ed), 291*(6488), 97-104. doi: 10.1136/bmj.291.6488.97

Medina-Leyte, D., Zepeda-García, O., Domínguez-Pérez, M., González-Garrido, A., Villarreal-Molina, T. & Jacobo-Albavera, L. (2021). Endothelial dysfunction, inflammation and coronary artery disease: Potential biomarkers and promising therapeutical approaches. *Int J Mol Sci, 22*(8), 3850. doi: 10.3390/ijms22083850

Melaku, Y., Reynolds, A., Appleton, S., Sweetman, A., Shi, Z., Vakulin, A., … Adams, R. (2022). High-quality and anti-inflammatory diets and a healthy lifestyle are associated with lower sleep apnea risk. *J Clin Sleep Med, 18*(6), 1667-1679. doi: 10.5664/jcsm.9950

Melguizo-Rodríguez, L., Costela-Ruiz, V., García-Recio, E., De Luna-Bertos, E., Ruiz, C. & Illescas-Montes, R. (2021). Role of Vitamin D in the Metabolic Syndrome. *Nutrients, 13*(3), 830. doi: 10.3390/nu13030830

Memon, A., Godward, S., Williams, D., Siddique, I. & Al-Saleh, K. (2010). Dental x-rays and the risk of thyroid cancer: a case-control study. *Acta Oncol, 49*(4), 447-53. doi: 10.3109/02841861003705778

Mendelsohn, R. (1982). How doctors manipulate women. Contemporary Books, Chicago

Menon, V., Kumar, A., Patel, D., St John, J., Riesmeyer, J., Weerakkody, G., … Nissen SE. Effect of CETP inhibition with evacetrapib in patients with diabetes mellitus enrolled in the ACCELERATE trial. *BMJ Open Diabetes Res Care, 8*(1), e000943. doi: 10.1136/bmjdrc-2019-000943

Michailidis, M., Moraitou, D., Tata, D., Kalinderi, K., Papamitsou, T. & Papaliagkas, V. (2022). Alzheimer's disease as type 3 diabetes: Common pathophysiological mechanisms between Alzheimer's disease and type 2 diabetes. *Int J Mol Sci, 23*(5), 2687. doi: 10.3390/ijms23052687

Millen, A., Tucker, M., Hartge, P., Halpern, A., Elder, D., Guerry, D. 4th., … Potischman, N. (2004). Diet and melanoma in a case-control study. *Cancer Epidemiol Biomarkers Prev, 13*(6), 1042-51

Miller, A., To, T., Baines, C. & Wall, C. (2000). Canadian National Breast Screening Study-2: 13-year results of a randomized trial in women aged 50-59 years. *J Natl Cancer Inst, 92*(18), 1490-9. doi: 10.1093/jnci/92.18.1490

Misciagna, G., Guerra, V., Di Leo, A., Correale, M. & Trevisan, M. (2000). Insulin and gall stones: a population case control study in southern Italy. *Gut, 47*(1), 144-7. doi: 10.1136/gut.47.1.144

Mlinarić, A., Horvat, M. & Šupak Smolčić, V. (2017). Dealing with the positive publication bias: Why you should really publish your negative results. *Biochem Med (Zagreb), 27*(3), 030201. doi: 10.11613/BM.2017.030201

Mohammadi-Sartang, M, Sohrabi, Z., Esmaeilinezhad, Z., Aqaeinezhad, R. & Jalilpiran, Y. (2018). Effect of conjugated linoleic acid on leptin level: A systematic review and meta-analysis of randomized controlled trials. *Horm Metab Res, 50*(2), 106-116. doi: 10.1055/s-0044-100041

Moore, M., Park, C. & Tsuda, H. (1998). Implications of the hyperinsulinaemia-diabetes-cancer link for preventive efforts. *Eur J Cancer Prev, 7*(2), 89-107

Moore, S., Carter, L. & van Goozen, S. (2009). Confectionery consumption in childhood and adult violence. *Br J Psychiatry, 195*(4), 366-7. doi: 10.1192/bjp.bp.108.061820

Mørch, L., Skovlund, C., Hannaford, P., Iversen, L., Fielding, S. & Lidegaard, Ø. (2017). Contemporary hormonal contraception and the risk of breast cancer. *N Engl J Med,377*(23), 2228-2239. Do i: 10.1056/NEJMoa1700732

Moskowitz, D. (2006). A comprehensive review of the safety and efficacy of bioidentical hormones for the management of menopause and related health risks. *Altern Med Rev, 11*(3), 208-23

Mozaffarian, D., Bryson, C., Lemaitre, R., Burke, G. & Siscovick, D. (2005). Fish intake and risk of incident heart failure. *J Am Coll Cardiol, 45*(12), 2015-21. doi: 10.1016/j.jacc.2005.03.038

Mozaffarian, D., Psaty, B., Rimm, E., Lemaitre, R., Burke, G., Lyles, M., … Siscovick, D. (2004). Fish intake and risk of incident atrial fibrillation. *Circulation, 110*(4), 368-73. doi: 10.1161/01.CIR.0000138154.00779.A5

Muldoon, M., Barger, S., Ryan, C., Flory, J., Lehoczky,

J., Matthews, K. & Manuck, S. (2000). Effects of lovastatin on cognitive function and psychological well-being. *Am J Med, 108*(7), 538-46. doi: 10.1016/s0002-9343(00)00353-3

Multiple risk factor intervention trial. Risk factor changes and mortality results. Multiple Risk Factor Intervention Trial Research Group. (1982) *JAMA, 248*(12):1465-77.

Naidoo, U. (2019). Nutritional psychiatry: the gut-brain connection. *Psychiatric times, 36*(1), 11A.

Nash, D., Magder, L., Lustberg, M., Sherwin, R., Rubin, R., Kaufmann, R. & Silbergeld, E. (2003). Blood lead, blood pressure, and hypertension in perimenopausal and postmenopausal women. *JAMA, 289*(12), 1523-32. doi: 10.1001/jama.289.12.1523

Navale, S., Mulugeta, A., Zhou, A., Llewellyn, D. & Hyppönen, E. (2022). Vitamin D and brain health: an observational and Mendelian randomization study. *Am J Clin Nutr, 116*(2), 531-540. doi: 10.1093/ajcn/nqac107

Navas-Acien, A., Guallar, E., Silbergeld, E. & Rothenberg, S. (2007). Lead exposure and cardiovascular disease--a systematic review. *Environ Health Perspect, 115*(3), 472-82. doi:

10.1289/ehp.9785

Navas-Acien, A., Selvin, E., Sharrett, A., Calderon-Aranda, E., Silbergeld, E. & Guallar, E. (2004). Lead, cadmium, smoking, and increased risk of peripheral arterial disease. *Circulation, 109*(25), 3196-201. doi: 10.1161/01.CIR.0000130848.18636.B2

Needleman, H., McFarland, C., Ness, R., Fienberg, S. & Tobin, M. (2002). Bone lead levels in adjudicated delinquents. A case control study. *Neurotoxicol Teratol, 24*(6), 711-7. doi: 10.1016/s0892-0362(02)00269-6

Neel, J. (1962). Diabetes mellitus: a "thrifty" genotype rendered detrimental by "progress"? *Am J Hum Genet, 14(4)*, 353-62

Ness, G. & Chambers, C. (2000). Feedback and hormonal regulation of hepatic 3-hydroxy-3-methylglutaryl coenzyme A reductase: the concept of cholesterol buffering capacity. *Proc Soc Exp Biol Med, 224*(1), 8-19. doi: 10.1046/j.1525-1373.2000.22359.x

Newman, T. & Hulley, S. (1996). Carcinogenicity of lipid-lowering drugs. *JAMA, 275*(1), 55-60

Ngo, A., Taylor, R., Roberts, C. & Nguyen, T. (2006). Association between Agent Orange and birth defects: systematic review and meta-analysis. *Int J Epidemiol,*

35(5), 1220-30. doi: 10.1093/ije/dyl038

Niazi, M., Galehdar, N., Jamshidi, M., Mohammadi, R. & Moayyedkazemi, A. (2020). A review of the role of statins in heart failure treatment. *Curr Clin Pharmacol, 15*(1), 30-37. doi: 10.2174/1574884714666190802125627

Nicolopoulou-Stamati, P., Hens, L. & Sasco, A. (2015). Cosmetics as endocrine disruptors: are they a health risk? *Rev Endocr Metab Disord, 16*(4), 373-83. doi: 10.1007/s11154-016-9329-4

Nichols, A., Ravenscroft, C., Lamphiear, D., Ostrander, L. Jr. (1976). Daily nutritional intake and serum lipid levels. The Tecumseh studdy. *Am J Clin Nutr, 29*(12),1384-92. doi: 10.1093/ajcn/29.12.1384

Nielsen, F., Hunt, C., Mullen, L. & Hunt, J. (1987). Effect of dietary boron on mineral, estrogen, and testosterone metabolism in postmenopausal women. *FASEB J, 1*(5), 394-7

Noubiap, J., Nansseu, J., Lontchi-Yimagou, E., Nkeck, J., Nyaga, U., Ngouo, A., … Bigna, J. (2022). Geographic distribution of metabolic syndrome and its components in the general adult population: A meta-analysis of global data from 28 million individuals. *Diabetes Res Clin Pract, 188*, 109924. doi:

10.1016/j.diabres.2022.109924

Nyström, L., Rutqvist, L., Wall, S., Lindgren, A., Lindqvist, M., Rydén, S., … Frisell, J., et al. (1993). Breast cancer screening with mammography: overview of Swedish randomised trials. *Lancet, 341*(8851), 973-8. doi: 10.1016/0140-6736(93)91067-v

Oba, S., Nanri, A., Kurotani, K., Goto, A., Kato, M., Mizoue, T., … Tsugane, S; Japan Public Health Center-based Prospective Study Group. (2013). Dietary glycemic index, glycemic load and incidence of type 2 diabetes in Japanese men and women: the Japan Public Health Center-based Prospective Study. *Nutr J, 12*(1), 165. doi: 10.1186/1475-2891-12-165

Okuyama, H., Langsjoen, P., Hamazaki, T., Ogushi, Y., Hama, R., Kobayashi, T. & Uchino, H. (2015). Statins stimulate atherosclerosis and heart failure: pharmacological mechanisms. *Expert Rev Clin Pharmacol, 8*(2), 189-99. doi: 10.1586/17512433.2015.1011125

Ono, A., Koshiyama, M., Nakagawa, M., Watanabe, Y., Ikuta, E., Seki, K.& Oowaki, M. (2020). The preventive effect of dietary antioxidants on cervical cancer development. *Medicina (Kaunas), 56*(11), 604. doi: 10.3390/medicina56110604

Ooi, S., Green, R. & Pak, S. (2018). N-Acetylcysteine

for the Treatment of Psychiatric Disorders: A Review of Current Evidence. *Biomed Res Int, 2018*, 2469486. doi: 10.1155/2018/2469486

Orlich, M., Mashchak, A., Jaceldo-Siegl, K., Utt, J., Knutsen, S., Sveen, L. & Fraser, G. (2022). Dairy foods, calcium intakes, and risk of incident prostate cancer in Adventist Health Study-2. *Am J Clin Nutr, 116*(2), 314-324. doi: 10.1093/ajcn/nqac093

Owens, J.; Adolescent Sleep Working Group; Committee on Adolescence. (2014) Insufficient sleep in adolescents and young adults: an update on causes and consequences. *Pediatrics, 134*(3), e921-32. doi: 10.1542/peds.2014-1696

Oxenkrug, G. (2013). Insulin resistance and dysregulation of tryptophan-kynurenine and kynurenine-nicotinamide adenine dinucleotide metabolic pathways. *Mol Neurobiol, 48*(2), 294-301. doi: 10.1007/s12035-013-8497-4

Padayatty, S., Riordan, H., Hewitt, S., Katz, A., Hoffer, L & Levine, M. (2006). Intravenously administered vitamin C as cancer therapy: three cases. *CMAJ, 174*(7), 937-42. doi: 10.1503/cmaj.050346

Palmer, N., Bakos, H., Fullston, T. & Lane, M. (2012). Impact of obesity on male fertility, sperm function and molecular composition. *Spermatogenesis, 2*(4), 253-263. doi: 10.4161/spmg.21362

Panchal, S., Wanyonyi, S. & Brown, L. (2017). Selenium, vanadium, and chromium as micronutrients to improve metabolic syndrome. *Curr Hypertens Rep, 19*(3),10. doi: 10.1007/s11906-017-0701-x

Paolisso, G. & Barbagallo, M. (1997). Hypertension, diabetes mellitus, and insulin resistance: the role of intracellular magnesium. *Am J Hypertens, 10*(3), 346-55. doi: 10.1016/s0895-7061(96)00342-1

Papakostas, G., Shelton, R., Zajecka, J., Etemad, B., Rickels, K., Clain, A., … Fava, M. (2012). L-methylfolate as adjunctive therapy for SSRI-resistant major depression: results of two randomized, double-blind, parallel-sequential trials. *Am J Psychiatry, 169*(12), 1267-74. doi: 10.1176/appi.ajp.2012.11071114

Papakostas, G., Mischoulon, D., Shyu, I., Alpert, J. & Fava, M. (2010). S-adenosyl methionine (SAMe) augmentation of serotonin reuptake inhibitors for antidepressant nonresponders with major depressive disorder: a double-blind, randomized clinical trial. *Am J Psychiatry, 167*(8), 942-8. doi: 10.1176/appi.ajp.2009.09081198

Parsaik, A., Singh, B., Murad, M., Singh, K.,

Mascarenhas, S., Williams, M., … Rummans, T. (2014). Statins use and risk of depression: a systematic review and meta-analysis. *J Affect Disord, 160*, 62-7. doi: 10.1016/j.jad.2013.11.026

Pasternak, R. (2002). The ALLHAT lipid lowering trial--less is less. *JAMA. 2002, 288*(23), 3042-4. doi: 10.1001/jama.288.23.3042

Pati, S., Irfan, W., Jameel, A., Ahmed, S. & Shahid, R. (2023). Obesity and Cancer: A Current Overview of Epidemiology, Pathogenesis, Outcomes, and Management. *Cancers (Basel), 15*(2), 485. doi: 10.3390/cancers15020485

Pauley, S. (2004). Lighting for the human circadian clock: recent research indicates that lighting has become a public health issue. *Med Hypotheses, 63*(4), 588-96. doi: 10.1016/j.mehy.2004.03.020

Peled, N., Kassirer, M., Shitrit, D., Kogan, Y., Shlomi, D., Berliner, A. & Kramer, M. (2007). The association of OSA with insulin resistance, inflammation and metabolic syndrome. *Respir Med, 101*(8), 1696-701. doi: 10.1016/j.rmed.2007.02.025

Pengelley, J. (2007). Jumbo ambulance for obese patients. *Adelaide Advertiser,* 10 March, 3.

Pescatello, L., Franklin, B., Fagard, R., Farquhar, W.,

Kelley, G. & Ray, C.; American College of Sports Medicine. American College of Sports Medicine position stand. (2004). Exercise and hypertension. *Med Sci Sports Exerc, 36*(3), 533-53. doi: 10.1249/01.mss.0000115224.88514.3a

Peteliuk, V., Rybchuk, L., Bayliak, M., Storey, K. & Lushchak, O. (2021) Natural sweetener *Stevia rebaudiana*: Functionalities, health benefits and potential risks. *EXCLI J, 20*, 1412-1430. doi: 10.17179/excli2021-4211

Petursson, H., Sigurdsson, J., Bengtsson, C., Nilsen, T. & Getz, L. (2012) Is the use of cholesterol in mortality risk algorithms in clinical guidelines valid? Ten years prospective data from the Norwegian HUNT 2 study. *J Eval Clin Pract, 18*(1), 159-68. doi: 10.1111/j.1365-2753.2011.01767.x

Pittas, A., Lau, J., Hu, F. & Dawson-Hughes, B. (2007). The role of vitamin D and calcium in type 2 diabetes. A systematic review and meta-analysis. *J Clin Endocrinol Metab, 92*(6), 2017-29. doi: 10.1210/jc.2007-0298

Plagemann, A., Harder, T., Kohlhoff, R., Rohde, W. & Dörner, G. (1997). Glucose tolerance and insulin secretion in children of mothers with pregestational IDDM or gestational diabetes. *Diabetologia, 40*(9),

1094-100. doi: 10.1007/s001250050792

Port, S., Garfinkel, A. & Boyle, N. (2000). There is a non-linear relationship between mortality and blood pressure. *Eur Heart J, 21*(20), 1635-8. doi: 10.1053/euhj.2000.2227

Powell, E., Smith-Taillie, L. & Popkin, B. (2016). Added sugars intake across the distribution of US children and adult consumers: 1977-2012. *J Acad Nutr Diet, 116*(10), 1543-1550.e1. doi: 10.1016/j.jand.2016.06.003

Purnell, J., Zinman, B., Brunzell, J.; DCCT/EDIC Research Group. (2013). The effect of excess weight gain with intensive diabetes mellitus treatment on cardiovascular disease risk factors and atherosclerosis in type 1 diabetes mellitus: results from the Diabetes Control and Complications Trial/Epidemiology of Diabetes Interventions and Complications Study (DCCT/EDIC) study. *Circulation, 127*(2), 180-7. doi: 10.1161/CIRCULATIONAHA.111.077487

Raitakari, O., Adams, M., McCredie, R., Griffiths, K. & Celermajer, D. (1999) Arterial endothelial dysfunction related to passive smoking is potentially reversible in healthy young adults. *Ann Intern Med, 130*(7), 578-81. doi: 10.7326/0003-4819-130-7-199904060-00017

Rajaraman, P., Simpson, J., Neta, G., Berrington de Gonzalez, A., Ansell, P., Linet, M., … Roman, E. (2011). Early life exposure to diagnostic radiation and ultrasound scans and risk of childhood cancer: case-control study. *BMJ, 342*, d472. doi: 10.1136/bmj.d472

Rapisarda, V., Miozzi, E., Loreto, C., Matera, S., Fenga, C., Avola, R. & Ledda, C. (2018). Cadmium exposure and prostate cancer: insights, mechanisms and perspectives. *Front Biosci (Landmark Ed), 23*(9), 1687-1700. doi: 10.2741/4667

Rathna, R., Varjani, S. & Nakkeeran, E. (2018). Recent developments and prospects of dioxins and furans remediation. *J Environ Manage, 223*, 797-806. doi: 10.1016/j.jenvman.2018.06.095

Ravdin, P., Cronin, K., Howlader, N., Berg, C., Chlebowski, R., Feuer, E., … Berry, D. (2007). The decrease in breast-cancer incidence in 2003 in the United States. *N Engl J Med, 356*(16), 1670-4. doi: 10.1056/NEJMsr070105

Ravnskov, U. (2002). Is atherosclerosis caused by high cholesterol? *QJM, 95*(6), 397-403. doi: 10.1093/qjmed/95.6.397

Ravnskov, U. (2008). The fallacies of the lipid hypothesis. *Scand Cardiovasc J, 42*(4), 236-9. doi: 10.1080/14017430801983082

Ravnskov, U., de Lorgeril, M., Diamond, D., Hama, R., Hamazaki, T., Hammarskjöld, B., … Sundberg R. (2018). LDL-C does not cause cardiovascular disease: a comprehensive review of the current literature. *Expert Rev Clin Pharmacol, 11*(10), 959-970. doi: 10.1080/17512433.2018.1519391

Raz, I., Karsai, D. & Katz, M. (1989). The influence of zinc supplementation on glucose homeostasis in NIDDM. *Diabetes Res, 11*(2), 73-9

Razay, G. & Wilcock, G. (1994). Hyperinsulinaemia and Alzheimer's disease. *Age Ageing, 23*(5), 396-9. doi: 10.1093/ageing/23.5.396

Reaven, G. & Hoffman, B. (1989). Hypertension as a disease of carbohydrate and lipoprotein metabolism. *Am J Med, 87*(6A), 2S-6S. doi: 10.1016/0002-9343(89)90488-9

Redberg, R. & Katz, M. (2017). Statins for Primary Prevention: The Debate Is Intense, but the Data Are Weak. *JAMA Intern Med,177*(1), 21-23. doi: 10.1001/jamainternmed.2016.7585

Reichman, M., Hayes, R., Ziegler, R., Schatzkin, A., Taylor. P., Kahle, L. & Fraumeni, J. Jr. (1990). Serum vitamin A and subsequent development of prostate cancer in the first National Health and Nutrition

Examination Survey Epidemiologic Follow-up Study. *Cancer Res, 50*(8), 2311-5

Rhee, S., Yon, D., Kwon, M., Kim, J., Kim, J., Bang, W., … Min C. (2022). Association between metabolic syndrome and osteoporosis among adults aged 50 years and older: using the National Health Information Database in South Korea. *Arch Osteoporos, 17*(1), 124. doi: 10.1007/s11657-022-01161-2

Ried, K. (2020). Garlic lowers blood pressure in hypertensive subjects, improves arterial stiffness and gut microbiota: A review and meta-analysis. *Exp Ther Med, 19*(2), 1472-1478. doi: 10.3892/etm.2019.8374

Rodríguez-Morán, M. & Guerrero-Romero, F. (2003). Oral magnesium supplementation improves insulin sensitivity and metabolic control in type 2 diabetic subjects: a randomized double-blind controlled trial. *Diabetes Care, 26*(4), 1147-52. doi: 10.2337/diacare.26.4.1147

Rondanelli, M., Faliva, M., Tartara, A., Gasparri, C., Perna, S., Infantino, V., … Peroni, G. (2021). An update on magnesium and bone health. *Biometals, 34*(4), 715-736. doi: 10.1007/s10534-021-00305-0

Rosenson, R. & Tangney, C. (1998). Antiatherothrombotic properties of statins: implications for cardiovascular event reduction. *JAMA, 279*(20),

1643-50. doi: 10.1001/jama.279.20.1643

Rossouw, J., Anderson, G., Prentice, R., LaCroix, A., Kooperberg, C., Stefanick, M., … Ockene, J; Writing Group for the Women's Health Initiative Investigators. (2002). Risks and benefits of estrogen plus progestin in healthy postmenopausal women: principal results From the Women's Health Initiative randomized controlled trial. *JAMA, 288*(3), 321-33. doi: 10.1001/jama.288.3.321

Roth, T. (2007). Insomnia: definition, prevalence, etiology, and consequences. *J Clin Sleep Med, 3*(5 Suppl), S7-10.

Roussel, A., Kerkeni, A., Zouari, N., Mahjoub, S., Matheau, J. & Anderson, R. (2003). Antioxidant effects of zinc supplementation in Tunisians with type 2 diabetes mellitus. *J Am Coll Nutr, 22*(4), 316-21. doi: 10.1080/07315724.2003.10719310

Rozati, R., Reddy, P., Reddanna, P. & Mujtaba, R. (2002). Role of environmental estrogens in the deterioration of male factor fertility. *Fertil Steril, 78*(6), 1187-94. doi: 10.1016/s0015-0282(02)04389-3

Russell, C., Baker, P., Grimes, C., Lindberg, R., & Lawrence, M. (2023). Global trends in added sugars and non-nutritive sweetener use in the packaged food supply: drivers and implications for public health. *Public Health Nutr, 26*(5), 952-964. doi: 10.1017/S1368980022001598

Ryan, T. & Shaw, C. (2015). Gracility of the modern Homo sapiens skeleton is the result of decreased biomechanical loading. *Proc Natl Acad Sci U S A, 112*(2), 372-7. doi: 10.1073/pnas.1418646112

Sahebzamani, F., D'Aoust, R., Friedrich, D., Aiyer, A., Reis, S. & Kip, K. (2013). Relationship among low cholesterol levels, depressive symptoms, aggression, hostility, and cynicism. *J Clin Lipidol, 7*(3), 208-16. doi: 10.1016/j.jacl.2013.01.004

Saher, G., Brügger, B., Lappe-Siefke, C., Möbius, W., Tozawa, R., Wehr, M., … Nave, K. (2005). High cholesterol level is essential for myelin membrane growth. *Nat Neurosci, 8*(4), 468-75. doi: 10.1038/nn1426

Saklayen, M. (2018). The global epidemic of the metabolic syndrome. *Curr Hypertens Rep, 20*(2), 12. doi: 10.1007/s11906-018-0812-z

Saleh, S., El-Kemery, T., Farrag, K., Badawy, M., Sarkis, N., Soliman, F. & Mangoud H. (2004). Ramadan fasting: relation to atherogenic risk among obese Muslims. *J Egypt Public Health Assoc, 79*(5-6), 461-83

Sales, C. & Pedrosa, L. (2006). Magnesium and diabetes mellitus: their relation. *Clin Nutr, 25*(4), 554-62. doi: 10.1016/j.clnu.2006.03.003

Sales, C., Pedrosa, L., Lima, J., Lemos, T. & Colli, C. (2011). Influence of magnesium status and magnesium intake on the blood glucose control in patients with type 2 diabetes. *Clin Nutr, 30*(3), 359-64. doi: 10.1016/j.clnu.2010.12.011

Salmerón, J., Ascherio, A., Rimm, E., Colditz, G., Spiegelman, D., Jenkins, D., … Willett, W. (1997). Dietary fiber, glycemic load, and risk of NIDDM in men. *Diabetes Care, 20*(4), 545-50. doi: 10.2337/diacare.20.4.545

Salmerón, J., Hu, F., Manson, J., Stampfe,r M., Colditz, G., Rimm, E., & Willett, W. (2001). Dietary fat intake and risk of type 2 diabetes in women. *Am J Clin Nutr, 73*(6), 1019-26. doi: 10.1093/ajcn/73.6.1019

Salmerón, J., Manson, J., Stampfer, M., Colditz, G., Wing, A., & Willett, W. (1997). Dietary fiber, glycemic load, and risk of non-insulin-dependent diabetes mellitus in women. *JAMA, 277*(6), 472-7. doi: 10.1001/jama.1997.03540300040031

Saremi, A., Bahn, G., Reaven, P.; VADT Investigators. (2012). Progression of vascular calcification is increased with statin use in the Veterans Affairs Diabetes Trial (VADT). *Diabetes Care, 35*(11), 2390-2. doi: 10.2337/dc12-0464

Sastry, K., Karpova, Y., Prokopovich, S., Smith, A., Essau, B., Gersappe, A., … Kulik G. (2007). Epinephrine protects cancer cells from apoptosis via activation of cAMP-dependent protein kinase and BAD phosphorylation. *J Biol Chem, 282*(19), 14094-100. doi: 10.1074/jbc.M611370200

Schandelmaier, S., Briel, M., Saccilotto, R., Olu, K., Arpagaus, A., Hemkens, L, & Nordmann, A. (2017). Niacin for primary and secondary prevention of cardiovascular events. *Cochrane Database Syst Rev, 6*(6), CD009744. doi: 10.1002/14651858.CD009744.pub2

Schatz, I., Masaki, K., Yano, K., Chen, R., Rodriguez, B. & Curb, J. (2001). Cholesterol and all-cause mortality in elderly people from the Honolulu Heart Program: a cohort study. *Lancet, 358*(9279), 351-5. doi: 10.1016/S0140-6736(01)05553-2

Schleifer, S., Keller, S., Camerino, M., Thornton, J. & Stein, M. (1983). Suppression of lymphocyte stimulation following bereavement. *JAMA, 250*(3), 374-7

Schoenthaler, S. & Bier, I. (2000). The effect of

vitamin-mineral supplementation on juvenile delinquency among American schoolchildren: a randomized, double-blind placebo-controlled trial. *J Altern Complement Med, 6*(1), 7-17. doi: 10.1089/acm.2000.6.7

Schott, G., Pachl, H., Limbach, U., Gundert-Remy, U., Lieb, K. & Ludwig, W. (2010). The financing of drug trials by pharmaceutical companies and its consequences: part 2: a qualitative, systematic review of the literature on possible influences on authorship, access to trial data, and trial registration and publication. *Dtsch Arztebl Int, 107*(17), 295-301. doi: 10.3238/arztebl.2010.0295

Schulze, M., Manson, J., Ludwig, D., Colditz, G., Stampfer, M., Willett, W., & Hu, F. (2004). Sugar-sweetened beverages, weight gain, and incidence of type 2 diabetes in young and middle-aged women. *JAMA, 292*(8), 927-34. doi: 10.1001/jama.292.8.927

Schutten, J., Joosten, M., de Borst, M. & Bakker, S. (2018). Magnesium and blood pressure: A physiology-based approach. *Adv Chronic Kidney Dis, 25*(3), 244-250. doi: 10.1053/j.ackd.2017.12.003

Scragg, R., Jackson, R., Holdaway, I., Lim, T. & Beaglehole, R. (1990). Myocardial infarction is inversely associated with plasma 25-hydroxyvitamin

D3 levels: a community-based study. *Int J Epidemiol, 19*(3), 559-63. doi: 10.1093/ije/19.3.559

See, K., Lavercombe, P., Dillon, J. & Ginsberg, R. (2006). Accidental death from acute selenium poisoning. *Med J Aust, 185*(7), 388-9. doi: 10.5694/j.1326-5377.2006.tb00616.x

Segoviano-Mendoza, M., Cárdenas-de la Cruz, M., Salas-Pacheco, J., Vázquez-Alaniz, F., La Llave-León, O., Castellanos-Juárez, F., … Méndez-Hernández, E. (2018). Hypocholesterolemia is an independent risk factor for depression disorder and suicide attempt in Northern Mexican population. *BMC Psychiatry, 18*(1):7. doi: 10.1186/s12888-018-1596-z

Sengupta, P. (2014). Current trends of male reproductive health disorders and the changing semen quality. *Int J Prev Med, 5*(1), 1-5.

Sephton, S, & Spiegel, D. (2003). Circadian disruption in cancer: a neuroendocrine-immune pathway from stress to disease? *Brain Behav Immun, 17*(5), 321-8. doi: 10.1016/s0889-1591(03)00078-3

Serrano Ríos, M. (2005). El síndrome metabólico: una versión moderna de la enfermedad ligada al estrés? [Metabolic syndrome: a modern variant of stress-related disease?]. *Rev Esp Cardiol, 58*(7), 768-71.

Spanish. doi: 10.1157/13077226

Sharpe, R. & Skakkebaek, N. (1993). Are oestrogens involved in falling sperm counts and disorders of the male reproductive tract? *Lancet, 341*(8857), 1392-5. doi: 10.1016/0140-6736(93)90953-e

Shaw, J. & Chisholm, D. (2003). 1: Epidemiology and prevention of type 2 diabetes and the metabolic syndrome. *Med J Aust, 179*(7), 379-83. doi: 10.5694/j.1326-5377.2003.tb05677.x

Sheehan, C., Frochen, S., Walsemann, K. & Ailshire, J. (2019). Are U.S. adults reporting less sleep?: Findings from sleep duration trends in the National Health Interview Survey, 2004-2017. *Sleep, 42*(2), zsy221. doi: 10.1093/sleep/zsy221

Sheldon, T. (2007). Television show questions statins to boost ratings, Dutch doctors claim. *BMJ, 334*(7594), 604-5. doi: 10.1136/bmj.39157.755718.DB

Shih, Y., Hung, C., Huang, C., Chou, K., Niu, S., Chan, S. & Tsai, H. (2020). The association between smartphone use and breast cancer risk among Taiwanese women: A case-control study. *Cancer Manag Res, 12*, 10799-10807. doi: 10.2147/CMAR.S267415

Shimada, B., Alfulaij, N. & Seale, L. (2021) The

impact of selenium deficiency on cardiovascular function. *Int J Mol Sci, 22*(19), 10713. doi: 10.3390/ijms221910713

Shiraseb, F., Asbaghi, O., Bagheri, R., Wong, A., Figueroa, A. & Mirzaei, K. (2022). Effect of l-arginine supplementation on blood pressure in adults: A systematic review and dose-response meta-analysis of randomized clinical trials. *Adv Nutr, 13*(4), 1226-1242. doi: 10.1093/advances/nmab155

Simopoulos, A & Robinson, J. (1998). *The Omega Plan*: Hodder and Stoughton, Australia

Simopoulos, A. (2002). The importance of the ratio of omega-6/omega-3 essential fatty acids. *Biomed Pharmacother, 56*(8), 365-79. doi: 10.1016/s0753-3322(02)00253-6

Singh, L., Sharma, S., Xu, S., Tewari, D. & Fang, J. (2021). Curcumin as a natural remedy for atherosclerosis: A pharmacological review. *Molecules, 26*(13), 4036. doi: 10.3390/molecules26134036

Singh, R., Chang, H., Yan, D., Lee, K., Ucmak, D., Wong, K., … Liao, W. (2017). Influence of diet on the gut microbiome and implications for human health. *J Transl Med, 15*(1), 73. doi: 10.1186/s12967-017-1175-y

Sismondo, S. (2021). Epistemic Corruption, the Pharmaceutical Industry, and the Body of Medical Science. *Front Res Metr Anal, 6*, 614013. doi: 10.3389/frma.2021.614013

Skaletz-Rorowski, A. & Walsh, K. (2003). Statin therapy and angiogenesis. *Curr Opin Lipidol, 14*(6), 599-603. doi: 10.1097/00041433-200312000-00008

Skallevold, H., Rokaya, N., Wongsirichat, N. & Rokaya, D. (2023). Importance of oral health in mental health disorders: An updated review. *J Oral Biol Craniofac Res, 13*(5), 544-552. doi: 10.1016/j.jobcr.2023.06.003

Soares, F., de Oliveira Matoso, R., Teixeira, L., Menezes, Z., Pereira, S., Alves, A., … Alvarez-Leite, J. (2013). Gluten-free diet reduces adiposity, inflammation and insulin resistance associated with the induction of PPAR-alpha and PPAR-gamma expression. *J Nutr Biochem, 24*(6), 1105-11. doi: 10.1016/j.jnutbio.2012.08.009

Sojka, J. & Weaver, C. (1995). Magnesium supplementation and osteoporosis. *Nutr Rev, 53*(3), 71-4. doi: 10.1111/j.1753-4887.1995.tb01505.x

Solga, S., Alkhuraishe, A., Clark, J., Torbenson, M., Greenwald, A., Diehl, A., Magnuson, T. (2004).

Dietary composition and nonalcoholic fatty liver disease. *Dig Dis Sci, 49*(10), 1578-83. doi: 10.1023/b:ddas.0000043367.69470.b7

Soliman, G. (2018) Dietary cholesterol and the lack of evidence in cardiovascular disease. *Nutrients, 10*(6), 780. doi: 10.3390/nu10060780

Sorrells, S., Caso, J., Munhoz, C. & Sapolsky, R. (2009). The stressed CNS: when glucocorticoids aggravate inflammation. *Neuron, 64*(1), 33-9. doi: 10.1016/j.neuron.2009.09.032

Spencer, H., Kramer, L., DeBartolo, M., Norris, C. & Osis, D. (1983). Further studies of the effect of a high protein diet as meat on calcium metabolism. *Am J Clin Nutr, 37*(6), 924-9. doi: 10.1093/ajcn/37.6.924

Spring, B. (1984). Recent research on the behavioral effects of tryptophan and carbohydrate. *Nutr Health, 3*(1-2), 55-67. doi: 10.1177/026010608400300204

Srour, B. & Touvier, M. (2021). Ultra-processed foods and human health: What do we already know and what will further research tell us? *EClinicalMedicine, 32*, 100747. doi: 10.1016/j.eclinm.2021.100747

Steegmans, P., Hoes, A., Bak, A., van der Does, E. & Grobbee, D. (2000). Higher prevalence of depressive symptoms in middle-aged men with low serum cholesterol levels. *Psychosom Med, 62*(2), 205-11. doi: 10.1097/00006842-200003000-00009

Stevens, R. (2006). Artificial lighting in the industrialized world: circadian disruption and breast cancer. *Cancer Causes Control, 17*(4), 501-7. doi: 10.1007/s10552-005-9001-x

Stewart, A. & Kneale, G. (1970). Radiation dose effects in relation to obstetric x-rays and childhood cancers. *Lancet, 1*(7658), 1185-8. doi: 10.1016/s0140-6736(70)91782-4

Strause, L., Saltman, P., Smith, K., Bracker, M. & Andon, M. (1994). Spinal bone loss in postmenopausal women supplemented with calcium and trace minerals. *J Nutr, 124*(7), 1060-4. doi: 10.1093/jn/124.7.1060

Suglia, S., Solnick, S. & Hemenway, D. (2013). Soft drinks consumption is associated with behavior problems in 5-year-olds. *J Pediatr, 163*(5), 1323-8. doi: 10.1016/j.jpeds.2013.06.023

Sungthong, B., Yoothaekool, C., Promphamorn, S. & Phimarn, W. (2020). Efficacy of red yeast rice extract on myocardial infarction patients with borderline hypercholesterolemia: A meta-analysis of randomized controlled trials. *Sci Rep, 10*(1), 2769. doi: 10.1038/s41598-020-59796-5

Susman, E., Dockray, S., Schiefelbein, V., Herwehe, S., Heaton, J. & Dorn, L. (2007). Morningness/eveningness, morning-to-afternoon cortisol ratio, and antisocial behavior problems during puberty. *Dev Psychol, 43*(4), 811-22. doi: 10.1037/0012-1649.43.4.811

Tabrizi, R., Akbari, M., Sharifi, N., Lankarani, K., Moosazadeh, M., Kolahdooz, F., … Asemi, Z. (2018). The effects of coenzyme Q10 supplementation on blood pressures among patients with metabolic diseases: A systematic review and meta-analysis of randomized controlled trials. *High Blood Press Cardiovasc Prev, 25*(1), 41-50. doi: 10.1007/s40292-018-0247-2

Taheri, S., Lin, L., Austin, D., Young, T. & Mignot, E. (2004). Short sleep duration is associated with reduced leptin, elevated ghrelin, and increased body mass index. *PLoS Med, 1*(3), e62. doi: 10.1371/journal.pmed.0010062

Talib, W., Alsayed, A., Abuawad, A., Daoud, S. & Mahmod, A. (2021). Melatonin in Cancer Treatment: Current Knowledge and Future Opportunities. *Molecules, 26*(9), 2506. doi: 10.3390/molecules26092506

Tarnowska, K., Gruczyńska-Sękowska, E., Kowalska,

D., Majewska, E., Kozłowska, M. & Winkler R. (2023). The opioid excess theory in autism spectrum disorders - is it worth investigating further? *Crit Rev Food Sci Nutr, 63*(19), 3980-3993. doi: 10.1080/10408398.2021.1996329

Tavani, A., Pregnolato, A., La Vecchia, C., Negri, E., Talamini, R. & Franceschi, S. (1997). Coffee and tea intake and risk of cancers of the colon and rectum: a study of 3,530 cases and 7,057 controls. *Int J Cancer, 73*(2), 193-7. doi: 10.1002/(sici)1097-0215(19971009)73:2<193::aid-ijc5>3.0.co;2-r

Taylor, K., Troester, M., Herring, A., Engel, L., Nichols, H., Sandler, D. & Baird, D. (2018). Associations between personal care product use patterns and breast cancer risk among white and black women in the sister study. *Environ Health Perspect, 126*(2), 027011. doi: 10.1289/EHP1480

Thomas, M., Blesso, C., Calle, M., Chun, O., Puglisi, M. & Fernandez, M. (2022). Dietary influences on gut microbiota with a focus on metabolic syndrome. *Metab Syndr Relat Disord, 20*(8), 429-439. doi: 10.1089/met.2021.0131

Thompson, K., Lichter, J., LeBel, C., Scaife, M., McNeill, J. & Orvig, C. (2009). Vanadium treatment of type 2 diabetes: a view to the future. *J Inorg Biochem,*

103(4), 554-8. doi: 10.1016/j.jinorgbio.2008.12.003

Till, C. & Green, R. (2021). Controversy: The evolving science of fluoride: when new evidence doesn't conform with existing beliefs. *Pediatr Res, 90*(5), 1093-1095. doi: 10.1038/s41390-020-0973-8

Titus-Ernstoff, L., Hatch, E., Hoover, R., Palmer, J., Greenberg, E., Ricker, W., … Hartge, P. (2001). Long-term cancer risk in women given diethylstilbestrol (DES) during pregnancy. *Br J Cancer, 84*(1),126-33. doi: 10.1054/bjoc.2000.1521

Titus, L., Hatch, E., Drake, K., Parker, S., Hyer, M., Palmer, J., … Troisi, R. (2019). Reproductive and hormone-related outcomes in women whose mothers were exposed in utero to diethylstilbestrol (DES): A report from the US National Cancer Institute DES Third Generation Study. *Reprod Toxicol, 84*, 32-38. doi: 10.1016/j.reprotox.2018.12.008

Tobi, E., Lumey, L., Talens, R., Kremer, D., Putter, H., Stein, A., … Heijmans, B. (2009). DNA methylation differences after exposure to prenatal famine are common and timing- and sex-specific. *Hum Mol Genet, 18*(21), 4046-53. doi: 10.1093/hmg/ddp353

Törnqvist, H., Mills, N., Gonzalez, M., Miller, M., Robinson, S., Megson, I., … Blomberg, A. (2007). Persistent endothelial dysfunction in humans after diesel exhaust inhalation. *Am J Respir Crit Care Med, 176*(4), 395-400. doi: 10.1164/rccm.200606-872OC

Treffers, P., Hanselaar, A., Helmerhorst, T., Koster, M. & van Leeuwen, F. (2001). Gevolgen van diëthylstilbestrol in de zwangerschap: na 50 jaar nog steeds een actueel probleem [Consequences of diethylstilbestrol during pregnancy; 50 years later still a significant problem]. *Ned Tijdschr Geneeskd, 145*(14), 675-80. Dutch.

Treviño, S. & Diaz, A. (2020). Vanadium and insulin: Partners in metabolic regulation. *J Inorg Biochem, 208*, 111094. doi: 10.1016/j.jinorgbio.2020.111094

Treviño, S., Díaz, A., Sánchez-Lara, E., Sanchez-Gaytan, B., Perez-Aguilar, J. & González-Vergara, E. (2019). Vanadium in biological action: Chemical, pharmacological aspects, and metabolic implications in diabetes mellitus. *Biol Trace Elem Res, 188*(1), 68-98. doi: 10.1007/s12011-018-1540-6

Trifiletti, L., Shields, W., Bishai, D., McDonald, E., Reynaud, F. & Gielen, A. (2006). Tipping the scales: obese children and child safety seats. *Pediatrics, 117*(4), 1197-202. doi: 10.1542/peds.2005-1379

Tsagari, A. (2020). Dietary protein intake and bone health. *J Frailty Sarcopenia Falls, 5*(1), 1-5. doi:

10.22540/JFSF-05-001

Tucker, K., Morita, K., Qiao, N., Hannan, M., Cupples, L. & Kiel, D. (2006). Colas, but not other carbonated beverages, are associated with low bone mineral density in older women: The Framingham Osteoporosis Study. *Am J Clin Nutr, 84*(4), 936-42. doi: 10.1093/ajcn/84.4.936

Vallverdú-Queralt, A., Jáuregui, O., Medina-Remón, A. & Lamuela-Raventós, R. (2012). Evaluation of a method to characterize the phenolic profile of organic and conventional tomatoes. *J Agric Food Chem, 60*(13), 3373-80. doi: 10.1021/jf204702f

Vancheri, F., Backlund, L., Strender, L., Godman, B. & Wettermark, B. (2016). Time trends in statin utilisation and coronary mortality in Western European countries. *BMJ Open, 6*(3), e010500. doi: 10.1136/bmjopen-2015-010500

Vasselli, J., Scarpace, P., Harris, R. & Banks, W. (2013). Dietary components in the development of leptin resistance. *Adv Nutr, 4*(2), 164-75. doi: 10.3945/an.112.003152

Venn, B. & Green, T. (2007). Glycemic index and glycemic load: measurement issues and their effect on diet-disease relationships. *Eur J Clin Nutr, 61* Suppl 1, S122-31. doi: 10.1038/sj.ejcn.1602942

Venniyoor, A. (2020). PTEN: A Thrifty Gene That Causes Disease in Times of Plenty? *Front Nutr, 7*, 81. doi: 10.3389/fnut.2020.00081

Vgontzas, A., Bixler, E. & Chrousos, G. (2005). Sleep apnea is a manifestation of the metabolic syndrome. *Sleep Med Rev, 9*(3), 211-24. doi: 10.1016/j.smrv.2005.01.006

Vidt, D. & Pohl, M. (1999). Aggressive blood pressure lowering is safe, but benefit is still hard to prove. *Cleve Clin J Med, 66*(2), 105-11. doi: 10.3949/ccjm.66.2.105

Vinceti, M., Filippini. T., Del Giovane, C., Dennert, G., Zwahlen, M., Brinkman, M., … Crespi, C. (2018). Selenium for preventing cancer. *Cochrane Database Syst Rev, 1*(1), CD005195. doi: 10.1002/14651858.CD005195.pub4

Vinogradova, Y., Coupland, C. & Hippisley-Cox, J. (2011). Exposure to statins and risk of common cancers: a series of nested case-control studies. *BMC Cancer, 11*, 409. doi: 10.1186/1471-2407-11-409

Vinogradova, Y., Coupland, C., Brindle, P. & Hippisley-Cox, J. (2016). Discontinuation and restarting in patients on statin treatment: prospective open cohort study using a primary care database. *BMJ, 353*, i3305. doi: 10.1136/bmj.i3305

Vorona, R., Winn, M., Babineau, T., Eng, B., Feldman, H., Ware, J. (2005). Overweight and obese patients in a primary care population report less sleep than patients with a normal body mass index. *Arch Intern Med, 165*(1), 25-30. doi: 10.1001/archinte.165.1.25

Walsh, J. & Pignone, M. (2004). Drug treatment of hyperlipidemia in women. *JAMA, 291*(18), 2243-52. doi: 10.1001/jama.291.18.2243

Wang, H., Yang, J., Qin, L. & Yang, X. (2015). Effect of garlic on blood pressure: a meta-analysis. *J Clin Hypertens (Greenwich), 17*(3), 223-31. doi: 10.1111/jch.12473

Wang, J., Xiong, X.& Feng, B. (2013). Effect of crataegus usage in cardiovascular disease prevention: an evidence-based approach. *Evid Based Complement Alternat Med, 2013*, 149363. doi: 10.1155/2013/149363

Wang, M., Yu, M., Fang, L. & Hu, R. (2015). Association between sugar-sweetened beverages and type 2 diabetes: A meta-analysis. *J Diabetes Investig, 6*(3), 360-6. doi: 10.1111/jdi.12309

Warner, M., Eskenazi, B., Mocarelli, P., Gerthoux, P, Samuels, S., Needham, L., … Brambilla, P. (2002). Serum dioxin concentrations and breast cancer risk in the Seveso Women's Health Study. *Environ Health Perspect, 110*(7), 625-8. doi: 10.1289/ehp.02110625

Watson, K., Simard, J., Henderson, V., Nutkiewicz, L., Lamers, F., Nasca, C., … Penninx B. (2021). Incident Major Depressive Disorder Predicted by Three Measures of Insulin Resistance: A Dutch Cohort Study. *Am J Psychiatry, 178*(10), 914-920. doi: 10.1176/appi.ajp.2021.20101479

Watson, G. & Craft, S. (2003). The role of insulin resistance in the pathogenesis of Alzheimer's disease: implications for treatment. *CNS Drugs, 17*(1), 27-45. doi: 10.2165/00023210-200317010-00003

Weeratunga, P., Jayasinghe, S., Perera, Y., Jayasena, G. & Jayasinghe, S. (2014). Per capita sugar consumption and prevalence of diabetes mellitus--global and regional associations. *BMC Public Health, 14*, 186. doi: 10.1186/1471-2458-14-186

Weiss, P., Scholz, H., Haas, J., Tamussino, K, Seissler, J. & Borkenstein, M. (2000). Long-term follow-up of infants of mothers with type 1 diabetes: evidence for hereditary and nonhereditary transmission of diabetes and precursors. *Diabetes Care, 23*(7), 905-11. doi: 10.2337/diacare.23.7.905

Welihinda, J., Karunanayake, E., Sheriff, M. & Jayasinghe, K. (1986). Effect of Momordica charantia on the glucose tolerance in maturity onset diabetes. *J Ethnopharmacol, 17*(3), 277-82. doi: 10.1016/0378-

8741(86)90116-9

Welty, F., Alfaddagh, A.& Elajami, T. (2016). Targeting inflammation in metabolic syndrome. *Transl Res, 167*(1), 257-80. doi: 10.1016/j.trsl.2015.06.017

West, J., Kapoor, N., Liao, S., Chen, J., Bailey, L. & Nagourney, R. (2013). Multifocal breast cancer in young women with prolonged contact between their breasts and their cellular phones. *Case Rep Med, 2013*, 354682. doi: 10.1155/2013/354682

Weverling-Rijnsburger, A., Blauw, G., Lagaay, A., Knook, D., Meinders, A, & Westendorp, R. (1997). Total cholesterol and risk of mortality in the oldest old. Lancet. 1997 Oct 18;350(9085):1119-23. doi: 10.1016/s0140-6736(97)04430-9

Whillier, S. (2020). Exercise and insulin resistance. *Adv Exp Med Biol, 1228*, 137-150. doi: 10.1007/978-981-15-1792-1_9

White, J. Jr. (2018). Sugar. *Clin Diabetes, 36*(1), 74-76. doi: 10.2337/cd17-0084

Whitmer, R., Gunderson, E., Barrett-Connor, E., Quesenberry, C. Jr. & Yaffe, K. (2005). Obesity in middle age and future risk of dementia: a 27 year longitudinal population based study. *BMJ, 330*(7504), 1360. doi: 10.1136/bmj.38446.466238.E0

Wiciński, M., Fajkiel-Madajczyk, A., Kurant, Z., Gryczka, K., Kurant, D., Szambelan, M., … Słupski, M. (2023). The use of cannabidiol in metabolic syndrome-An opportunity to improve the patient's health or much ado about nothing? *J Clin Med, 12*(14), 4620. doi: 10.3390/jcm12144620

Willett, W., Manson, J. & Liu, S. (2002). Glycemic index, glycemic load, and risk of type 2 diabetes. *Am J Clin Nutr, 76*(1), 274S-80S. doi: 10.1093/ajcn/76/1.274S

Wolfe, R. (2000). Effects of insulin on muscle tissue. *Curr Opin Clin Nutr Metab Care, 3*(1), 67-71. doi: 10.1097/00075197-200001000-00011

Wolraich, M., Wilson, D. & White, J. (1995). The effect of sugar on behavior or cognition in children. A meta-analysis. *JAMA, 274*(20), 1617-21. doi: 10.1001/jama.1995.03530200053037

Woodruff, T. & Walker, C. (2008). Fetal and early postnatal environmental exposures and reproductive health effects in the female. *Fertil Steril, 89*(2 Suppl), e47-51. doi: 10.1016/j.fertnstert.2007.12.029

World Health Organization. (2003). *Diet, nutrition and the prevention of chronic diseases.* Geneva: WHO.

Wright, C. & Mueller, C. (1995). Screening

mammography and public health policy: the need for perspective. *Lancet 346*(8966), 29-32. doi: 10.1016/s0140-6736(95)92655-0.

Wright, J., Lanphear, B., Dietrich, K., Bolger, M., Tully, L., Cecil, K. & Sacarellos, C. (2021). Developmental lead exposure and adult criminal behavior: A 30-year prospective birth cohort study. *Neurotoxicol Teratol, 85*, 106960. doi: 10.1016/j.ntt.2021.106960

Wu, Y., Dong, Y., Duan, S., Zhu, D. & Deng, L. (2017). Metabolic Syndrome, *Inflammation, and Cancer, 8259356*. doi: 10.1155/2017/8259356

Xiao, Q., Garaulet, M. & Scheer, F. (2019). Meal timing and obesity: interactions with macronutrient intake and chronotype. *Int J Obes,* 43, 1701–1711, doi: 10.1038/s41366-018-0284-x

Xu, P., Liu, A., Li, F., Tinkov, A., Liu, L. & Zhou, J. (2021). Associations between metabolic syndrome and four heavy metals: A systematic review and meta-analysis. *Environ Pollut, 273*, 116480. doi: 10.1016/j.envpol.2021.116480

Xu, Z., McClure, S. & Appel, L. (2018). Dietary Cholesterol Intake and Sources among U.S Adults: Results from National Health and Nutrition Examination Surveys (NHANES), 2001‑2014.

Nutrients, 10(6), 771. doi: 10.3390/nu10060771

Yaggi, H., Araujo, A. & McKinlay, J. (2006). Sleep duration as a risk factor for the development of type 2 diabetes. *Diabetes Care, 29*(3), 657-61. doi: 10.2337/diacare.29.03.06.dc05-0879

Yam, D., Eliraz, A. & Berry, E. (1996). Diet and disease--the Israeli paradox: possible dangers of a high omega-6 polyunsaturated fatty acid diet. *Isr J Med Sci, 32*(11), 1134-43

Yamaguchi, M., Eguchi, M., Akter, S., Kochi, T., Hu, H., Kashino, I., … Mizoue, T. (2018). The association of work-related stressors and their changes over time with the development of metabolic syndrome: The Furukawa Nutrition and Health Study. *J Occup Health, 60*(6):485-493. doi: 10.1539/joh.2017-0298-OA

Yan, H., Chen, Y., Zhu, H., Huang, W., Cai, X., Li, D., … Li, X. (2022). The Relationship Among Intestinal Bacteria, Vitamin K and Response of Vitamin K Antagonist: A Review of Evidence and Potential Mechanism. *Front Med (Lausanne),* 9, 829304. doi: 10.3389/fmed.2022.829304

Yang, J., Li, C., Shen, Y., Zhou, H., Shao, Y., Zhu, W. & Chen, Y. (2020). Impact of statin use on cancer-specific mortality and recurrence: A meta-analysis of

60 observational studies. *Medicine (Baltimore), 99*(14), e19596. doi: 10.1097/MD.0000000000019596

Yates, K., Sweat, V., Yau, P., Turchiano, M. & Convit, A. (2012). Impact of metabolic syndrome on cognition and brain: a selected review of the literature. *Arterioscler Thromb Vasc Biol, 32*(9), 2060-7. doi: 10.1161/ATVBAHA.112.252759

Yuan, R., Yuan, Y., Wang, L., Xin, Q., Wang, Y., Shi, W., … Cong, W; and BPNMI Consortium. (2022). Red Yeast Rice Preparations Reduce Mortality, Major Cardiovascular Adverse Events, and Risk Factors for Metabolic Syndrome: A Systematic Review and Meta-analysis. *Front Pharmacol, 13*, 744928. doi: 10.3389/fphar.2022.744928

Zeiher, A, Schächinger, V. & Minners, J. (1995). Long-term cigarette smoking impairs endothelium-dependent coronary arterial vasodilator function. *Circulation, 92*(5), 1094-100. doi: 10.1161/01.cir.92.5.1094

Zhang, A., Xia, Y., Lin, J., Chu, K., Wang, W., Ruiter, T., … Kopp, J. (2023). Hyperinsulinemia acts via acinar insulin receptors to initiate pancreatic cancer by increasing digestive enzyme production and inflammation. *Cell Metab. 2023 Oct 26*, S1550-4131(23)00372-8. doi: 10.1016/j.cmet.2023.10.003

Zhang, H., Plutzky, J., Skentzos, S., Morrison, F., Mar,

P., Shubina, M. & Turchin, A. (2013). Discontinuation of statins in routine care settings: a cohort study. *Ann Intern Med, 158*(7), 526-34. doi: 10.7326/0003-4819-158-7-201304020-00004

Zhang, J., Muldoon, M., McKeown, R. & Cuffe, S. (2005). Association of serum cholesterol and history of school suspension among school-age children and adolescents in the United States. *Am J Epidemiol, 161*(7), 691-9. doi: 10.1093/aje/kwi074

Zhang, J., Cai, A., Chen, G., Wang, X., Cai, M., Li, H., … Lin, H. (2022). Habitual fish oil supplementation and the risk of incident atrial fibrillation: findings from a large prospective longitudinal cohort study. *Eur J Prev Cardiol, 29*(14), 1911-1920. doi: 10.1093/eurjpc/zwac192

Zhang, X., Dai, B., Zhang, B. & Wang, Z. (2012). Vitamin A and risk of cervical cancer: a meta-analysis. *Gynecol Oncol, 124*(2), 366-73. doi: 10.1016/j.ygyno.2011.10.012

Zhang, Y., Yang, S., Wu, Q., Ye, Z., Zhou, C., Liu, M., … Qin, X. (2023). Dietary vitamin E intake and new-onset hypertension. *Hypertens Res, 46*(5), 1267-1275. doi: 10.1038/s41440-022-01163-0

Zhao, D., Liang, Y., Dai, S., Hou, S., Liu, Z., Liu, M.,

… Yang, Y. (2022). Dose-response effect of coenzyme Q10 supplementation on blood pressure among patients with cardiometabolic disorders: A grading of recommendations assessment, development, and evaluation (GRADE) assessed systematic review and meta-analysis of randomized controlled trials. *Adv Nutr, 13*(6), 2180-2194. doi: 10.1093/advances/nmac100

Zhao, J., Xu, L., Sun, J., Song, M., Wang, L., Yuan, S., … Li, X. (2023). Global trends in incidence, death, burden and risk factors of early-onset cancer from 1990 to 2019. *BMJ Oncology, 2*, e000049. doi: 10.1136/bmjonc-2023-000049

Zhelyazkova-Savova, M., Yotov, Y., Nikolova, M., Nazifova-Tasinova, N., Vankova, D., Atanasov, A. & Galunska, B. (2021). Statins, vascular calcification, and vitamin K-dependent proteins: Is there a relation? *Kaohsiung J Med Sci, 37*(7), 624-631. doi: 10.1002/kjm2.12373

Zittermann, A. (2003). Vitamin D in preventive medicine: are we ignoring the evidence? *Br J Nutr, 89*(5), 552-72. doi: 10.1079/BJN2003837

Zittermann, A. (2006). Vitamin D and disease prevention with special reference to cardiovascular disease. *Prog Biophys Mol Biol, 92*(1), 39-48. doi:

10.1016/j.pbiomolbio.2006.02.001

Zou, X., Sun, L., Yang, W., Li, B. & Cui, R. (2020). Potential role of insulin on the pathogenesis of depression. *Cell Prolif, 53*(5), e12806. doi: 10.1111/cpr.12806

Dr Peter Baratosy MBBS FACNEM

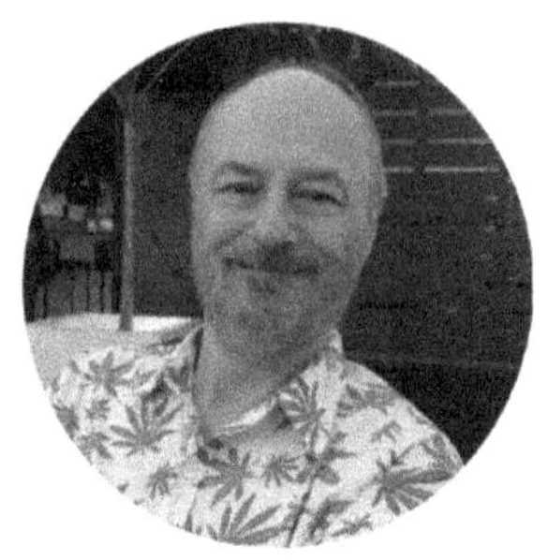

About Peter Baratosy

Peter Baratosy MBBS, FACNEM is a medical doctor, lecturer, and writer on chronic diseases, especially thyroid disease, gut disorders, hormonal problems and metabolic syndrome. Most recently he has written and published a book on CBD Oil. He has a great interest in using a more natural approach in treating chronic disease, though he does also use conventional medicines if, and when, needed. He graduated more than 40 years ago from the University of Adelaide Medical School in Australia and has over 35 years' experience as a functional medicine practitioner. He is a Fellow of the Australasian College of Nutritional and Environmental Medicine and is an accredited Medical Acupuncturist with the Medical Board of Australia. He lives in Tasmania with his wife Jenny.

www.ingramcontent.com/pod-product-compliance
Lightning Source LLC
Chambersburg PA
CBHW021841020426
42334CB00013B/147

* 9 7 8 0 6 4 5 1 0 5 3 7 7 *